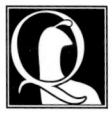

BEST OF THE BEST PRESENTS

# Instant LOW CARB

### FRESH KETO-FRIENDLY RECIPES FOR INSTANT POT® & ALL ELECTRIC PRESSURE COOKERS

### George Stella & Christian Stella

**QUAIL RIDGE PRESS**
*Preserving America's Food Heritage*

# QUAIL RIDGE PRESS

Copyright © 2019 George Stella

All rights reserved. No part of this book may be reproduced or transmitted in any form or by any means, electronic or mechanical, including photocopying or recording, or by any information retrieval system, without the written permission of the copyright holder.

This book is not meant to dispense medical advice. Please consult your doctor before making any dramatic changes to what you eat.

Instant Pot® is a registered trademark of Instant Brands Inc. The authors and publisher are not affiliated with or endorsed by Instant Brands Inc. Use of the words Instant Pot® without the registered trademark symbol ® is only done for the sake of legibility.

Nutritional analysis provided on each recipe is meant only as a reference and has been compiled to the best of our ability using nutritional analysis software. Due to differences in sizes, brands, and types of ingredients, your calculations may vary. Calories have been rounded to the nearest 5, and all other amounts were rounded to the nearest .5 of a gram.

Authors: George Stella and Christian Stella
Book design and food photography: Christian and Elise Stella
Proofreading and index: Linda Brock
Front cover: Instant Pot Roast, page: 115

Library of Congress Control Number: 2019930303

ISBN: 978-0-937552-05-6
Printed in the United States of America
10 9 8 7 6 5 4 3 2 1

(Best of the Best presents) *Instant Low Carb* was edited, designed, and manufactured by Quail Ridge Press. Quail Ridge Press is an imprint of Southwestern Publishing Group, Inc., 2451 Atrium Way, Nashville, TN 37214. Southwestern Publishing Group is a wholly owned subsidiary of Southwestern/Great American, Inc., Nashville, Tennessee.

Christopher G. Capen, President, Southwestern Publishing Group
Kristin Connelly, Managing Editor, Southwestern Publishing Group
Kristin Stephany, Director of Partner Development, Southwestern Publishing Group
Gwen and Barney McKee, Cofounders, Quail Ridge Press
Sheila Thomas, Publisher, Quail Ridge Press

quailridge.com | info@quailridge.com | 800-343-1583

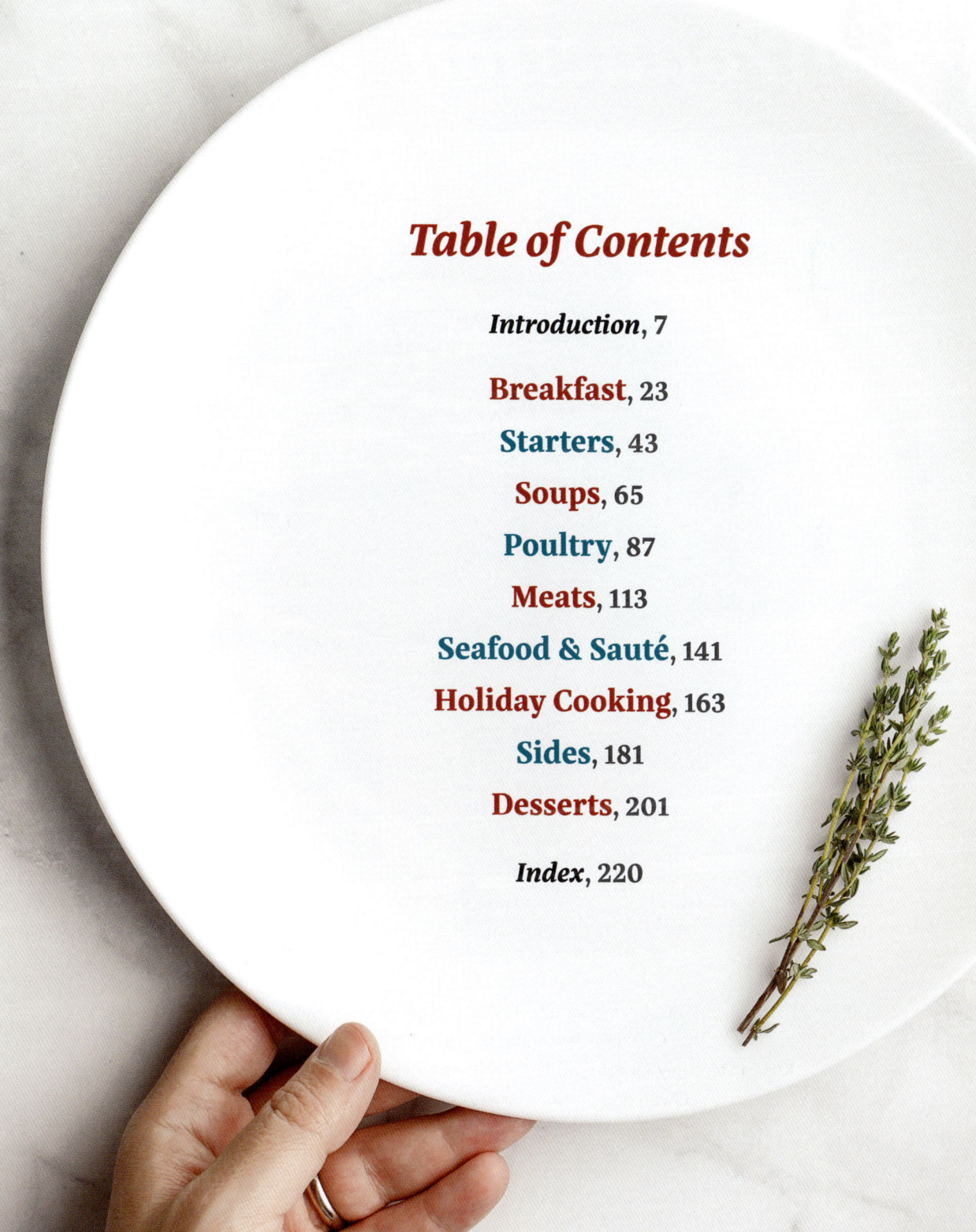

# Table of Contents

***Introduction***, 7

**Breakfast**, 23

**Starters**, 43

**Soups**, 65

**Poultry**, 87

**Meats**, 113

**Seafood & Sauté**, 141

**Holiday Cooking**, 163

**Sides**, 181

**Desserts**, 201

***Index***, 220

# *Introduction*

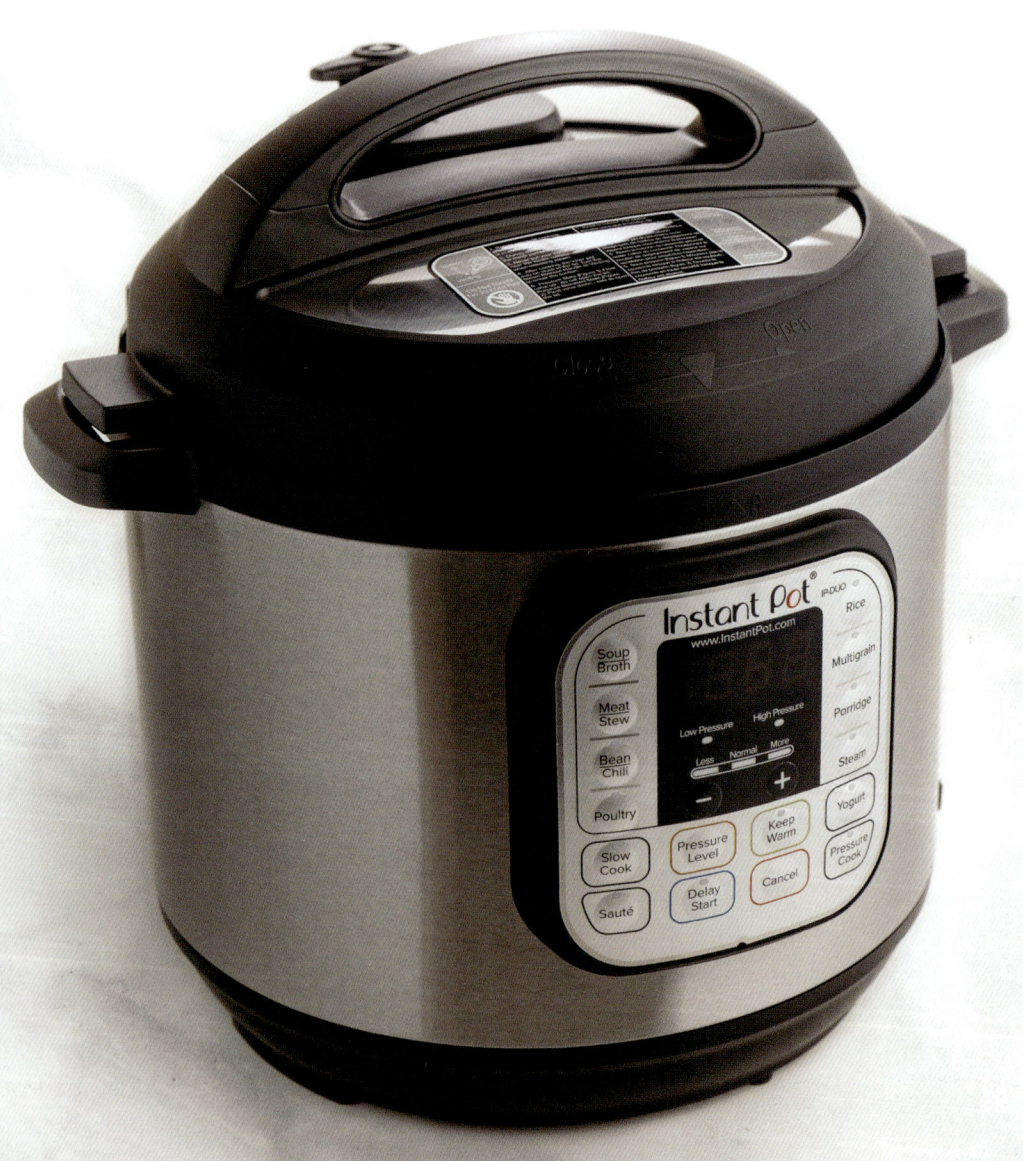

Whether you are already in love with your Instant Pot or are a new "Potter" joining our ever-increasing ranks, we hope you're excited to start cooking fresh, low-carb foods in a fraction of the time. The Instant Pot is truly changing how we cook in the kitchen and for how long!

We've been using electric pressure cookers like the Instant Pot for over a decade. Christian has even co-authored and done the food photography for two of the most popular pressure-cooking cookbooks of all time (alongside Bob Warden). Since then, he's worked with pressure cooker manufacturers on various projects. He's even done some food photography for Instant Pot's official site.

However, it wasn't until the recent increase in Instant Pot's awareness that there were enough cookers in people's homes for us to finally dedicate an entire low-carb cookbook to this method of cooking.

It only makes sense that this, our tenth cookbook, is the first book that we've fully co-authored together with equal credit, as father and son. The expert in low-carb and the expert in cooking under pressure. Our years of experience combining to help you cook delicious meals in an Instant—without all the carbs!

Twenty years ago, we were both obese—George weighing 467 pounds and Christian weighing 305 at only age fifteen. We were a "fat family" of four with mom, Rachel, and son Anthony also significantly overweight. Once a chef in the best restaurants in Florida, George was in a wheelchair with a myriad of weight-related ailments. We found out about low-carb at the exact right moment—when both our health and our spirits were failing.

### George and Christian, before

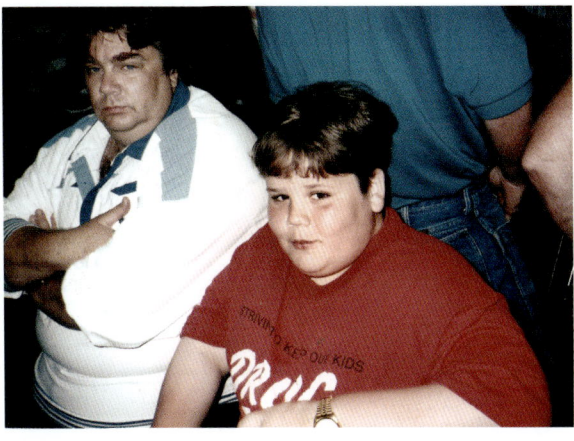

We had tried to "diet" in the past, but nothing ever stuck until low-carb. It was a plan that was more realistic and that didn't require us to give up ALL food, just those foods that were high in carbohydrates. It didn't leave us hungry, and more importantly, it actually worked.

Within three years, we had both lost more than half of our body weight—George down 265 pounds and Christian down 160. The entire family had lost a total of 560 pounds by living a low-carb lifestyle, and our health and spirits returned.

It began the next chapter of our lives, becoming champions for this simple and all-natural way of eating. We continue to maintain our weight loss by creating new recipes to keep things fresh and reinventing classics that we've been eating since we first started this journey. This book contains a combination of both new and classic dishes, reimagined and cooked in the Instant Pot for the very first time.

Losing weight is never easy, but low-carb was our easiest path to results. One of the biggest struggles with healthy eating is to find the time to cook for yourself without relying on takeout or delivery. The Instant Pot can help alleviate some of this struggle by cooking meals in far less time and without having to stand over them to supervise.

Instant Low Carb • 7

George and Rachel, after

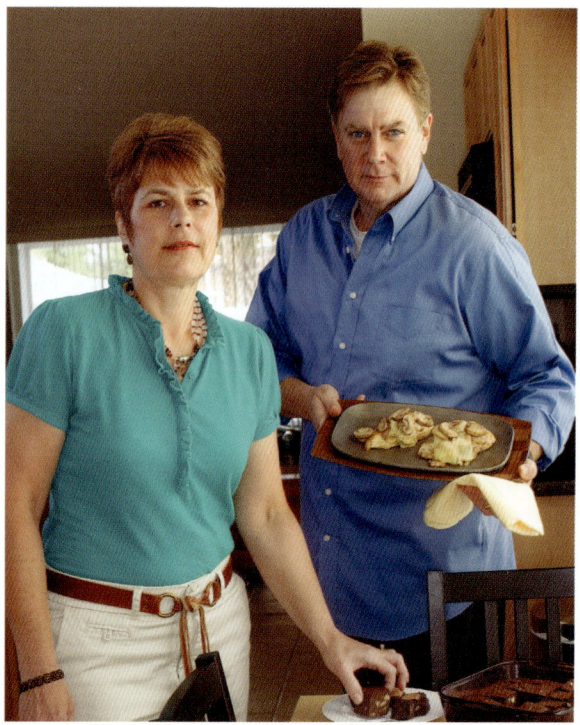

## The Basics of Low-Carb

The concept of eating low-carb is actually quite simple to explain. Our bodies are capable of converting either carbohydrates or fat into the energy needed to function; however, our bodies prefer carbohydrates when they are available. Eating a diet full of carbohydrates causes the body to burn only the carbs necessary to get through the day before then converting the remaining carbohydrates into fat, which is then stored—alongside the actual fat you eat—in the event there ever comes a time when excess fat is needed for survival. This is the reason that overeating leads to weight gain. When eating an abundance of carbs alongside fat, we store both as fat.

Your body can also create energy from fat when it is not supplied with an ample amount of carbohydrates. By converting fat into energy, your body goes into a constant fat-burning state known as "ketosis." Not only do you burn the fat that you eat, you can also burn through your reserved fat. Most people find it hard to grasp why low-carb allows you to eat fattier foods. There's a simple explanation: your body burns it right off.

Entering the "ketosis" state is easily achieved: simply stop eating processed carbohydrates. If you are looking to lose weight, staying in a state of ketosis is important to success. Cheating on a low-carb lifestyle will take your body out of ketosis and stop burning fat.

We refer to low-carb as a "lifestyle," as it works best when you eliminate processed carbohydrates completely, without cheating. This is how you achieve ketosis full-time for the maximum benefit.

If you have weight to lose, we suggest you fully embrace the low-carb lifestyle to hopefully start seeing the same benefits that we've seen. That said, we are not doctors, and you should always consult a doctor before making any changes to the way you eat.

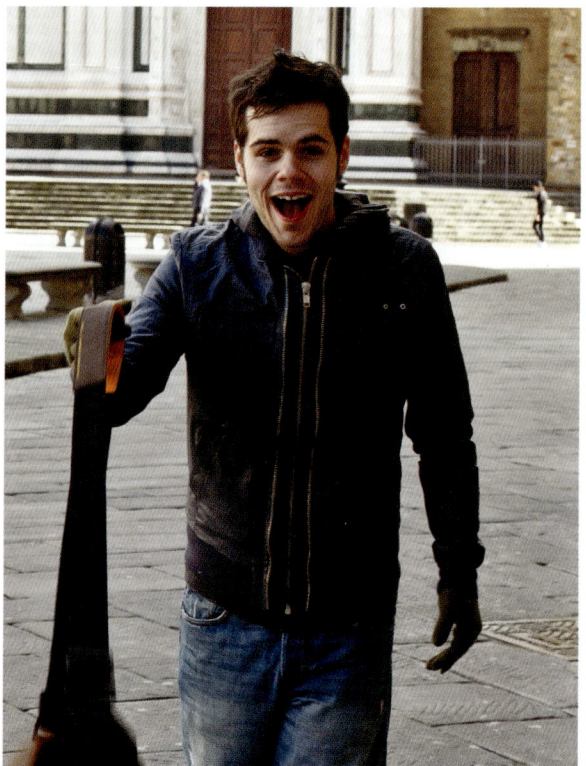

Christian, after

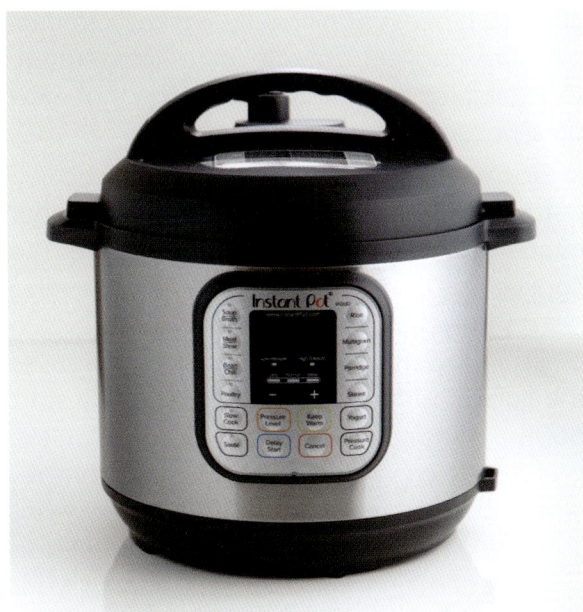

This valve must be closed (set to Sealing) for the pot to come up to pressure. The valve will usually jiggle, but that is completely normal, as it is a "floating" mechanism that uses the built-up pressure to stay closed.

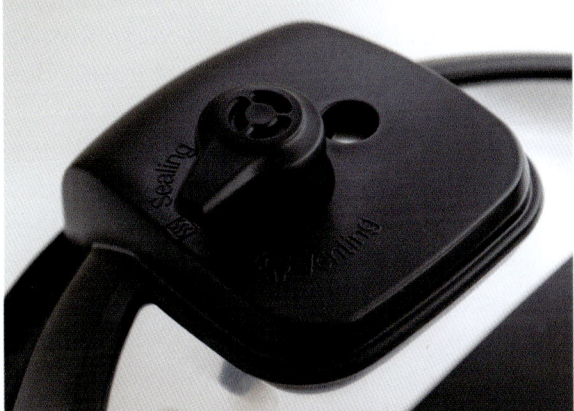

## The Basics of the Instant Pot

The Instant Pot and all electric pressure cookers have a removable inner pot that is seated inside of the main cooker.

Regardless of what you are cooking, some liquid must be added to convert to steam and create pressure inside the pot. This will vary depending on the type of food, but you will usually need at least $1/2$ cup of liquid. Some foods that contain a lot of natural liquid could get by with less but only because they will release some of that liquid as the cooker heats up and the food begins to cook.

The cooker's lid must be properly placed and (usually) twisted to lock over the pot. A silicone seal on the bottom of the lid ensures that no steam can escape from the connection between the pot and lid.

A valve on the top of the lid has two positions labeled:

1. **Venting** (open)
2. **Sealing** (closed)

The inner pot and the entire lid assembly are dishwasher safe. Most parts of the lid can be disassembled for deeper cleaning.

Once you've locked and sealed the lid, you can set your cook time using the buttons or dial on the front of your model of Instant Pot. The pot will then slowly come up to pressure. Once it has reached pressure, it will begin to count down the cook time that you entered.

Once the cook time has elapsed, the pressure must be safely released. There are two ways to do this:

1. **Quick Release** – Open the valve on the top of the lid by twisting to the "venting" position. This must be done very carefully, as it will immediately result in a very large blast of hot steam that may take over a minute to slow to a stop.

2. **Natural Release** – To let the pressure release naturally, you simply wait. The pressure will slowly reduce as the cooker cools down, until eventually it is safe to open. This can take anywhere from 5 to 30 minutes, though it most often takes 15.

Instant Low Carb • 9

We most often use a combination of both release methods by letting the pressure release naturally for a set period of time before quick releasing whatever smaller amount of pressure is left.

A floating steel indicator (a little smaller than a dime) to the side of the venting valve will drop once pressure is fully released. It is then safe to open the cooker.

While it may seem a bit daunting at first, this all becomes second nature in day to day operation. It is also comforting to know that unlike pressure cookers our grandmothers may have had growing up, the Instant Pot and other electric pressure cookers have a redundancy of safety features built into almost every part of the machine.

That said, you should always read and follow the manual that came with your particular model of cooker to ensure you are operating and properly maintaining the device as intended by the manufacturer.

## How it Actually Works

While it may seem like magic, Instant Pots and all electric pressure cookers turn liquid into steam and then use that steam to pressurize a sealed pot. Pressure increases to about 12 pounds per square inch or "psi" for short. With this amount of pressure, water doesn't boil until it reaches a much higher temperature than traditional cooking methods.

To understand why the boiling point of water is important, you must first know that boiling water stays a constant 212°F and does not get any hotter as it cooks, it simply begins the process of evaporation. This is even true for the water within food itself. You can cook a piece of meat at 400°F, but the water content of that meat will not go past the boiling point.

In the Instant Pot, water can get 30°F hotter before it begins to boil. This speeds up the cooking process significantly. Typically, electric pressure cookers operate at a temperature that ensures they stay just under that new pressurized boiling point.

Don't worry, your food isn't actually boiling inside the cooker, but it is cooking at a higher temperature than boiling water outside of the cooker. This is why opening the pressure valve results in so much steam: the sudden loss in pressure lowers the boiling point and causes the liquid inside the pot to immediately start boiling. When deciding between a "quick" pressure release or a "natural" pressure release, it's extremely helpful to picture what is happening inside the pot: a quick release is a sudden and immediate boiling of your food. For tender meat that can stand up to a long cook time, it is best to wait at least some amount of time before releasing the pressure.

## The Right Setting for the Job

When you first start using an Instant Pot, it can be very exciting to try to cook everything under pressure, whether you should be cooking that ingredient in that manner or not. We are not including pressure-cooked recipes for ingredients we would not cook under pressure in our day to day lives.

Once you factor in the time it takes for the pot to come up to pressure, the cook time, then the release time, a 1-minute shrimp recipe has become 12 minutes just to yield you results that may be overcooked. Just because you can doesn't always mean you should! Sautéing shrimp can yield perfect results that you can cook in around half the time of that same "1-minute" recipe.

The good news is that the Instant Pot does have a SAUTÉ setting, and it can be very convenient to use for easier cleanup, times when the stove is occupied, or even just because you really love that new Instant Pot!

This setting has allowed us to put a few more recipes in this book (in the Seafood & Sauté section) with more variety than just the ingredients we'd cook under pressure. We've included a few seafood recipes, one-pot skillet meals, and delicate vegetable side dishes that are too easily overcooked under pressure. It just didn't feel like a Stella-family cookbook without shrimp recipes!

## The True Cook Time

A common complaint about Instant Pot recipes is that they try to hide a dirty secret about pressure cooking: the time it takes the pot to come up to pressure. As we touched on in the previous section, it isn't an insignificant amount of time. All pressure cookers can take anywhere from 5 to 15 minutes to reach pressure and start the actual cook time's countdown. After that, many recipes will have a natural release period that increases the time even more.

We do not include the time it takes the pot to reach pressure—not to hide that time but to ensure that the numbers you need to see are easy to find at the top of the page. When you go to set your cooker, you can find the exact number you need to set without having to skim back through the directions. When it has finished cooking, you can find which type of release and the length of a natural pressure release. Times at the top of a page are meant as a quick reference for those situations—not the total cooking time.

It is our concern that if we were to include the time it takes to reach pressure within the cook time, some people may accidentally set their cooker to that total time and overcook the dish.

When cooking under pressure, always account for about 10 minutes of additional time for the pot to pressurize. There is still a huge time savings overall for most meat dishes and there are other benefits to pressure cooking (infusing flavors being the big one) for other ingredients that do not take as long to cook using traditional methods.

## The 0-Minute Cook Time

Some recipes in this book have a 0-minute cook time. This is not a typo and is actually a really great feature of the Instant Pot. When set to 0 minutes, the pot comes up to full pressure and then immediately shuts off. This allows you to cook delicate foods using only the time it takes to come up to pressure, or a combination of that and some amount of natural release. It's an especially good trick for quick-pickling vegetables without losing all of their crunch.

## Different Models and Sizes

The recipes in this book were tested using a 6-quart Instant Pot Duo. This is the most popular size and model of Instant Pot. That said, Christian has a decade of experience with different brands of electric pressure cookers of all different sizes—from 4-quart to 8-quart.

Recipes in this book can scale to an 8-quart cooker without issue. The only real downside of an 8-quart model is that it may take longer to build up the initial pressure (as there's more space inside the pot to pressurize).

Recipes will also work in a 4-quart cooker; however, you may need to cut or trim larger pieces of meat. You should also keep a close eye on the max-fill line, as many recipes will come very close to reaching it and variances in ingredient size will play a larger role in whether everything can fit. If you are ever above the line, simply use a ladle to remove some of the liquid.

The smallest "mini" models are not recommended but will certainly work for smaller recipes in this book. Other recipes will have to be halved, while still ensuring enough liquid is added to come to pressure.

## Other Brands of Pressure Cookers

Many brands have been selling electric pressure cookers for many, many years. Functionally, they are all extremely similar to the Instant Pot for cooking under pressure. While the recipes may mention "Instant Pot" by name, they can be prepared in any electric pressure cooker.

We've been making some of the most demanding recipes in this book for a decade with 4 different brands of cookers, and they've all taken the same amount of time under HIGH pressure. That said, we really do prefer the manual settings and quality of the Instant Pot.

Some brands of cookers may not allow you to set a manual temperature or time without hitting a programmed button and then adjusting that time. When in doubt, hit the "meat" or "beef" button and then adjust the time to match the recipe, as any meat setting will be that machine's highest level of pressure.

Some brands of cookers may not let you set them for a 0-minute cook time. For these recipes, you may need to set the cooker for 1 minute and then manually cancel the cooking process as soon as things have reached pressure. It's the simplest solution.

Be sure to read any cooker's instruction manual from front to back and familiarize yourself with their settings and guidelines and with how to safely operate their pressure-releasing valve.

Stovetop pressure cookers can reach a higher pressure level than electric pressure cookers and are not recommended for the cook times in this book. That said, if you are very familiar with your stovetop cooker, you may be able to prepare many of these recipes with small adjustments.

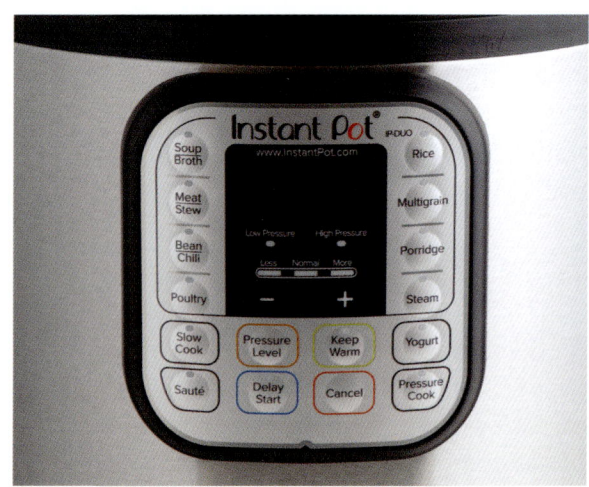

## Programmed Buttons

It is likely that your Instant Pot or pressure cooker has an array of pre-programmed buttons, however, this book makes use of only a few basic settings that can be found on any electric pressure cooker.

Buttons that are programmed to specific foods or dishes (such as meats, soups, etc.) can be convenient when you are cooking without a recipe, but their programming may differ from model to model and may change with future models. They are also only programmed to be as universal as they can be and are not smart enough to know exactly what you've put into the pot. These buttons should be ignored when cooking recipes from this book, as our cook times will be more accurate for our specific recipes.

Many pressure cookers have settings for either HIGH or LOW pressure. Low pressure can be helpful when cooking delicate foods like vegetables or seafood; however, we have developed and tested our recipes to use only the high-pressure setting. We made this decision because some very popular models of

Instant Pot simply do not have a low-pressure setting! We want to ensure that everyone can enjoy every recipe in the book without having to upgrade their cooker.

The only other function we use in this book is the SAUTÉ function to brown or cook food with the lid off. On some cookers, this may be labeled "BROWN." Your cooker may also have varying levels of power for the SAUTÉ button. Many models of Instant Pot have three levels (LESS, NORMAL, and MORE). We only use the highest level at all times. A lower setting is good for reheating a dish, but most often, you are using this setting to either brown something or bring a liquid up to a simmer, so you will want the most power.

**You should check your cooker to ensure it is set to the highest level when pressing SAUTÉ.** The Instant Pot does remember the settings you last used, and it is very easy to overlook that it may be set to "LESS" power.

The KEEP WARM function isn't mentioned in the recipes in this book, but it can be helpful for keeping a dish warm while entertaining or waiting for everyone to get to the table. We usually turn it off when we set the pressure-cooking time before cooking to ensure it doesn't keep the food warm during a natural pressure release, as that could add a small amount of time to how long the pressure takes to release. We've accidentally left it on as well, and it doesn't really seem to affect much.

**Please note:** Your Instant Pot may have a dial to select different settings but should be functionally identical to models that have dedicated buttons.

## Browning Meats

There seem to be two distinct groups among pressure-cooking fanatics:

1. Those who brown meat, sauté aromatics, and broil final dishes to enhance color and flavor.
2. Those who just want to throw it all in the pot, set the time, and have dinner ready in minutes because they are far too busy to fuss with all that other stuff.

Neither group is right or wrong, and both ways of approaching pressure cooking have their pluses and minuses. The "browning" group is adding a small amount of color and flavor at the expense of time, and the "set it and forget it" group is saving time at the expense of a small amount of color and flavor.

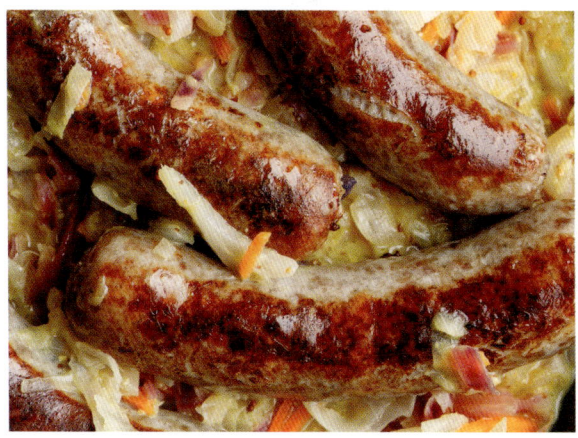

The recipes in this book have mostly been developed and written with the browning group in mind. This is how we cook, and this is the style of cooking that creates the better final dish. As cooking professionals, this is how we are *supposed* to cook even if it isn't always how we have *time* to cook. Whenever we found that it didn't add anything substantial, our recipes skip the browning and sautéing steps. Most often though, we do add extra steps of browning, sautéing, reducing, or broiling and it is all in the service of flavor. We are not trying to waste your time!

That said, you can often skip these steps. That choice is truly yours. If you've already been pressure cooking without browning and are happy with your results, you don't need to follow our recipes to the letter. There are only a few things that we find you should always brown:

- Ground meats, as they need to be crumbled before being added to liquid
- Chicken skin, as it gets rubbery and pale without it (you can remove it)
- Bacon, as it will also get rubbery

Onions and garlic will be sweeter and milder when sautéed before pressure cooking. Throwing them straight into the pot can sometimes overpower a dish with their raw flavor. But you may like those flavors! It is a bit silly that we all sauté onions to cook out their raw flavor when preparing a chili, then top that chili with raw onions! If you are going to skip the browning steps, we'd recommend reducing the amount of garlic and onions added by $1/2$ to ensure they don't overpower the dish.

## A Crowded Pot

When browning meats, the Instant Pot can get crowded. When the pot is crowded, it has a hard time getting hot enough to actually brown the meat. The meat will then release water, which will start boiling the meat—the exact opposite effect of what you're looking for! There are a few ways to fix this:

- Brown/sauté on the stove in a larger skillet over a higher heat than your cooker can reach. However, this does defeat the purpose of a multi-cooker by creating dishes and heating up the kitchen. It will likely give you the greatest results but is not ideal.

- Brown meat in smaller batches. We see this recommended a lot, but to be honest, no one wants to do this. It takes up a ton of time and also creates dishes as you transfer batches in and out of the cooker.
- If you are going to crowd the meat, push things to one side, ensuring that there is a good amount of empty (and hot) surface area for juices to evaporate rather than collect. This is the most realistic way to brown in such a small space. Leave some of the surface completely open, even if that means you have to pile things up on the other side.

## Preventing Stuck Food

When browning, some foods love to stick to the Instant Pot's stainless-steel inner pot. This is especially true of chicken, ground chicken or turkey, and seafood. There are a few ways to ensure this doesn't happen:

- Make sure there is oil across the entire bottom of the pot. The curvature of the pot can sometimes let it pool around the edges, requiring a little bit more oil to get to the center.
- Preheat the pot before adding the oil, then heat the oil until sizzling hot. Set the cooker to SAUTÉ and let stand for 3 minutes before adding the oil (this prevents the oil from burning as the pot heats). Many Instant Pots will actually display "HOT" on their display once the pot has preheated. Once preheated, add the oil and heat for at least 30 seconds before adding the food.
- Order an official nonstick inner pot for the Instant Pot. It really helps with poultry and seafood! Plus, having a second pot allows you to cook a dish while the other pot is in the dishwasher or fridge.

# Building Flavors

For many, pressure cooking is an entirely new way of cooking, which may take some adjustments—both literally and figuratively. When cooking under pressure, flavors are built and develop differently than traditional methods of sautéing, braising, grilling, or baking.

Many people prefer the way flavors mellow out and infuse into the food while cooking under pressure, but others may find that the flavors aren't as easily identifiable as they are used to. When the flavors meld, you may miss the contrast or brightness of traditional cooking methods. Acid, salt, herbs, and spices will all taste subtler when cooked under pressure.

While you can't open the cooker to taste and adjust seasonings once pressurized, this does not mean that you can't or shouldn't build flavors before serving. There are a few ways that this can be done after cooking:

- Reduce the cooking liquid by switching the cooker to SAUTÉ and bringing up to a simmer until the flavors have increased in strength to your liking.
- Add a splash of acid (vinegar, citrus juice, wine) to brighten the overall flavor, especially if there was acid used in the recipe before cooking.
- Add a pinch of the same herbs or spices that were used in the recipe before cooking to add a second layer of their flavors.
- Drain some cooking liquid before adding the final ingredients. We do this often in our recipes, as sometimes more liquid is required or released when cooking than you need. By draining some of this cooking liquid, any cream, butter, cheese, or other finishing ingredient you add will get less watered down.
- Add an extra teaspoon of bouillon bases. The natural liquid in many ingredients can water down a dish, but a dab of chicken or beef base can really punch the flavor back up.
- Add a pinch of sugar substitute. A tiny hint of sweetness will bring out the salt in the dish without having to add additional salt.
- Season with salt and pepper to taste. We always adjust the amount of salt and pepper one last time before serving, even if they were added earlier in the cooking process.

We usually use at least two of these methods to adjust everything we cook in the Instant Pot before serving but your tastes may vary.

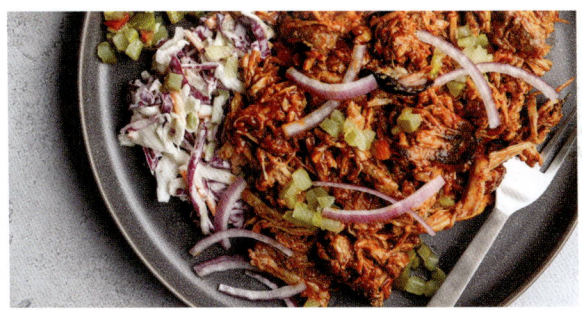

## Flavor Fixes

**If over-reduced or the dish is too salty:** Add water or fat in the form of oil, butter, or cream.

**If the dish is too acidic:** You can start by bringing the dish up to a simmer to cook some of the acid out. Add a pinch of sugar substitute to offset it with sweetness or add a pinch of baking soda, which will foam up and dissolve the acid. The baking soda can really mellow out the flavor of canned tomato products, removing some of that metallic aftertaste.

**If the dish is too sweet:** Add acid, salt, or fat, or simply water it down.

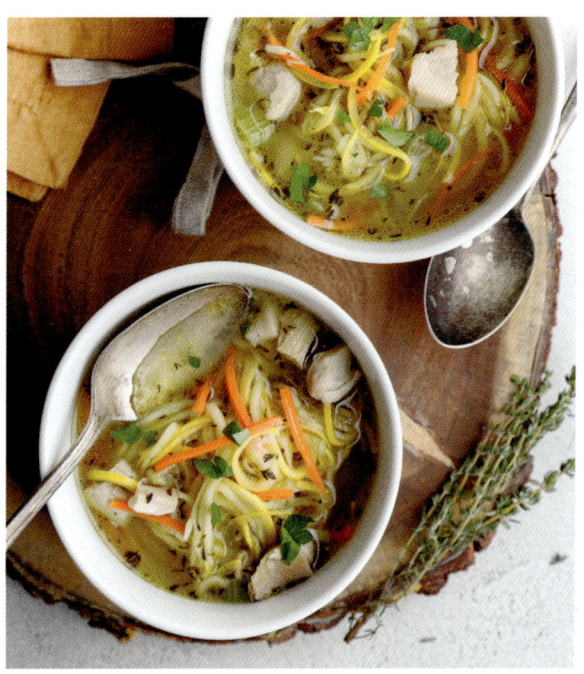

## Stocks and Broths

You will see us using beef, chicken, or vegetable stocks throughout most of the recipes in this book. As the Instant Pot requires some amount of liquid to build pressure, there is no reason to not add flavor as you add that liquid. It's a chef's trick!

We've chosen to recommend "stock," as stock is usually more flavorful than "broth," but either will work. Look for a brand with the least amount of carbs.

Concentrated bases will save you money (and shelf space) in the long run, as a small jar can make gallons of stock when dissolved in water. You can find them near the cartons of stock/broth in the grocery store. The bad news is that the most popular brands contain a very small amount of added sugar, so you will have to determine if that is acceptable on your eating plan.

Recipes that use a very small amount of stock ($1/2$ cup or less) can usually be made with water in a pinch. The impact on flavor will be negligible.

## Thickening Soups and Sauces

Thickening soups and sauces can be difficult on low-carb. Without the use of starch, some liquids may be thinner than you are used to, especially any kind of gravy. The good news is that this doesn't impact flavor! There are a few very low-carb options for thickeners and a few that will add some carbs and should only be used if they fit into your way of eating.

### Reducing

While it won't actually thicken the liquid that much, bringing a liquid up to a simmer and reducing it by evaporating some of the water will concentrate the flavors, which will ensure that it doesn't need to fully coat the dish to impart that flavor. If the dish includes tomatoes or certain vegetables, their natural starch will help thicken things as the liquid reduces.

### Heavy Cream

Adding heavy cream after pressure cooking will make any sauce or soup smoother, creamier, and more satisfying. Reducing the heavy cream will thicken it, but not to the levels that starchy thickeners will thicken it.

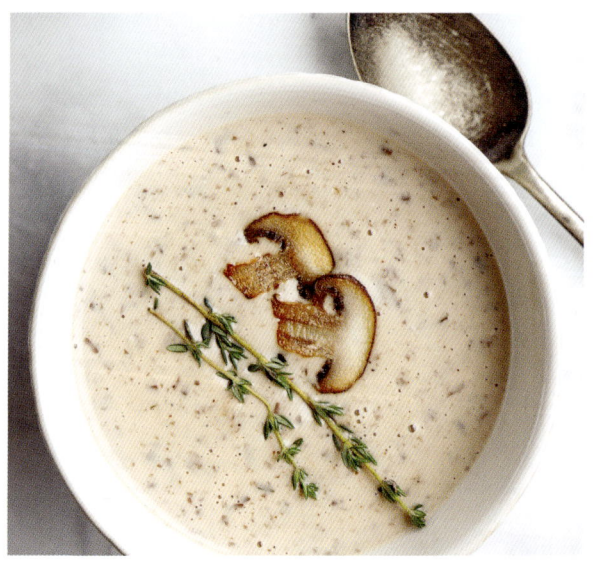

### Butter

When added after cooking, with the cooker off, butter will slightly thicken a sauce while making it more velvety smooth. For the best results, reduce liquids before adding the butter.

### Cream Cheese

Cream cheese will naturally thicken liquids somewhat better than heavy cream or butter. Stir it into a hot liquid with the cooker off to prevent burning. It is easier to incorporate the cream cheese into the liquid if you cut it into smaller pieces first. It will likely take a minute of stirring to fully incorporate it into the liquid. Whenever stirring it into liquids without large chunks of food in them, use a whisk to make your life easier!

### Puréed Cauliflower

Cooked and food-processed cauliflower makes a great thickener. This also works with broccoli stalks, so don't throw them away when cutting the florets from the bunch.

### Xanthan Gum

Many people on low-carb swear by the use of xanthan gum to thicken, but we've found it difficult to work with. You can usually find it in the gluten-free baking section of the store, or wherever you'd find almond flour. The total carbs seem bad at first, but it is almost entirely fiber, making the net carbs around 0. It should be lightly sprinkled over a liquid and then whisked or blended until smooth. A little goes a long way! For the best results, transfer some of the cooking liquid to a blender to blend with the gum until very thick, then use that mixture to thicken the rest of the dish.

### Arrowroot Starch

Sometimes referred to as "arrowroot powder," this is definitely a starch and isn't suitable for extremely carb-restricted diets. It is suitable for some low-carb plans, such as Paleo. This will all depend on how many and which types of carbs you want to be eating. A tablespoon of arrowroot starch is enough to thicken a meal for 6 people and contains 7g of carbs, so you are looking at only a little more than 1g of carbs per serving. It is used exactly as you'd use cornstarch. You whisk it into a very small amount of cold water before stirring into a simmering liquid to thicken.

### Cornstarch

Nutritionally and functionally, cornstarch is almost identical to the arrowroot starch above, even in carb counts. It absolutely can be an option for people who are only moderately watching their carbs, especially because so little is needed to thicken. The reason most health-conscious people prefer arrowroot starch is that cornstarch has links to corn that has been genetically modified (GMO). To avoid GMOs, arrowroot starch is the more natural choice.

## Accessorize Your Cooker

Many of the recipes in this book require additional accessories to prepare. Thanks to the popularity of the Instant Pot, these accessories are now extremely easy to find, especially online. You should have seen Christian trying to find a cheesecake pan for a 4-quart pressure cooker a decade ago! Many sellers online now sell all-in-one accessory packs that include most of these items for a reasonably low price. Some accessories may have even come with your cooker.

### Steam Rack

The steam rack will likely be your most-used accessory, and the manufacturer must know that, as all current cookers include one. This metal rack will allow you to elevate food above the cooking liquid to steam or even "bake" without directly coming in contact with the water or the cooker's heating element.

A good steam rack will have handles that unfold to allow you to lower and lift the rack in and out of the cooker. This is especially helpful for cake pans that are nearly the same width as the cooker, as those leave very little room for your hands to keep hold of the pan.

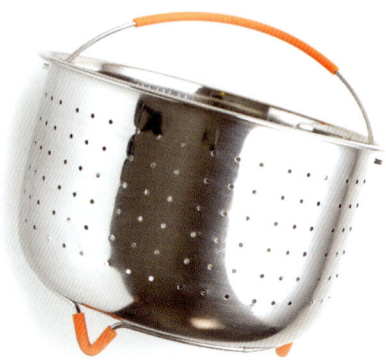

## Steam Basket

While many vegetables can be stacked up atop the steam rack, a steam basket is more convenient for smaller pieces or larger quantities. Unlike a steam rack, a basket is like a second pot within your Instant Pot, allowing you to remove and drain an entire basket of vegetables in one go.

There are two popular varieties of steam baskets.

A solid basket in the shape of a pot that may be made of wire mesh or stainless steel.

A collapsible disc-shaped basket that expands to fit any size pot. You may already own one of these for steaming on the stovetop.

Of the two, we prefer the first option as they are typically taller and have handles that are easier to grab. Most have silicone handles as well, which is nice when reaching into a hot cooker.

## Glass Lid

Instant Pot sells an official glass lid to fit their inner pots, but we found that we already had more than one glass lid that already fit! You may have a lid for a slow cooker or saucepot that fits as well.

This can be handy for using the SLOW COOK setting or heating ingredients on the SAUTÉ setting. The standard Instant Pot lid with pressure valve should not be used on these settings or it will try to build pressure.

## Ramekins

We use a set of four standard 4-ounce ramekins in several recipes in this book. These round ceramic dishes are great for making small baked goods or eggs. You can also use heatproof glass (such as Pyrex) custard cups. Depending on the thickness of the ceramic/glass, you may or may not be able to fit all four inside a 6-quart cooker in one layer. If you cannot, place three dishes in a triangular pattern and top with the fourth dish where those intersect.

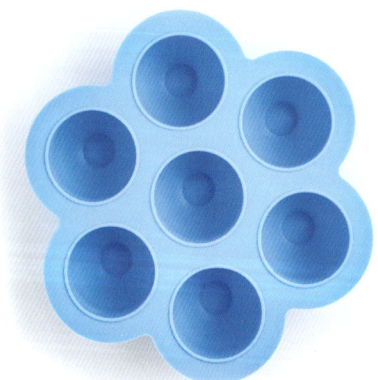

## Silicone Egg Bites Mold

Egg bites (like mini quiches) are becoming an Instant Pot phenomenon, but you'll need one of these silicone molds to make them. You can get them for a very reasonable price from a multitude of sellers online. Not just for eggs, we love to use this to make desserts!

### 7-inch Springform Pan

A must for Instant Pot "baking," springform pans are in two pieces, allowing you to unlock and remove the sides without damaging your baked goods. Most of the pans you will find in stores will start at 8 inches, which is a little too large to fit into the Instant Pot, but thankfully there are plenty of options online.

**Please note:** Springform pans are notorious for leaking if they are not tightly clasped. Under pressure, they have a somewhat opposite issue; steam can push its way into the pan where the two pieces meet. For this reason, you should always wrap the entire pan in aluminum foil (not just the top) before cooking.

### 7-inch Cake Pans

You can get away with using your springform pan exclusively, but we also like to have traditional cake pans as well, as they are one single piece and do not have the potential to leak. These can be especially handy for stacking on top of each other to cook two separate things at once.

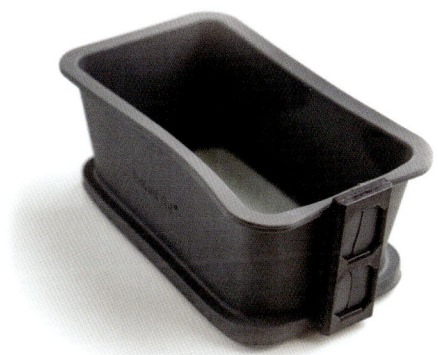

### 6.5-inch Loaf Pan

A small loaf pan can come in handy for certain desserts. We use a springform silicone loaf pan made by Instant Pot. It's a bit finnicky to put it together and take it apart and needs to be well-wrapped with aluminum foil.

### Nonstick Inner Pot

Instant Pot sells a nonstick inner pot that you can use in place of the stainless-steel pot that comes standard. It isn't necessary to own, but it can make cleanup a bit easier and will also help when browning foods that love to stick (seafood and some poultry).

If you are using your Instant Pot a few times a week, this one is a no-brainer, as a second inner pot will ensure you always have a clean cooker at your disposal. They even sell silicone lids to use your inner pots as storage containers in the fridge!

### Silicone Sealing Rings

This one is definitely a luxury, but you can buy additional silicone sealing rings for the bottom of the Instant Pot's lid. These are the gaskets that seal the lid shut to keep in the pressure. They are often sold in multiple packs with assorted colors to allow you to use set colors for the types of dishes you are cooking. This is because the silicone ring can retain the fragrance of many herbs and spices. If you have both a savory ring and a sweet ring, you won't have to worry about a dessert that has a faint taste of thyme or chicken with a hint of cinnamon.

We would only recommend buying the official Instant Pot sealing rings, as this piece is so integral to the cooker's operation.

### A Dry Dish Towel

It's a good habit to place a dry dish towel over the pressure vent when opening it to release the pressure. This will catch the steam before it can rise and collect on your kitchen cabinets and walls!

Many companies sell little attachments to redirect the steam, but then you'll just have the steam angled somewhere else in your kitchen, rather than into a simple towel that you already own.

Instant Low Carb • 19

## The Accessory You Shouldn't Use!

Every brand of pressure cooker we've ever purchased (including the Instant Pot) has come with a small plastic measuring cup. Put it away. Forget about it. You will not need it for this book and should not need it on a low-carb lifestyle. These measuring cups are always Asian rice measuring cups. They usually do not mention this in the instruction manual either. For whatever reason, 1 rice cup is only equal to about ¾ of an actual cup!

Beyond that, the measuring lines inside the removable inner pot of many electric pressure cookers (not the Instant Pot) are also meant for cooking rice and are not standard.

Using these measurements for any recipe (not just in this book) may cause the ratios to be wrong. It may even result in not adding enough liquid to bring the pot up to pressure. You are best off gifting the cup to someone who makes a lot of rice. You can also gift them a batch of cauliflower rice!

## Foods to Avoid on Low-Carb

You can't succeed on low-carb if you don't know which high-carb foods to avoid. Refined grains, sugars, and starches—otherwise known as "the white stuff"—are not a part of a low-carb lifestyle. This includes:

- Flour and all wheat products
- Sugars (including honey/syrups)
- Rice and similar grains
- White potatoes and potato products
- Corn
- High-sugar fruits and juice (bananas, mangos, grapes, watermelon, etc.)
- Beans
- Milk (cream is fine, but milk has more lactose, which is a form of sugar)

## About Nutritional Information

The nutritional analysis provided at the bottom of our recipes is meant only as a reference. It was compiled to the best of our ability using nutritional analysis software. Due to variances in the sizes of vegetables, brands of certain foods, or fat content of meat, calculations may vary.

Calculations are for each serving of the finished dish. Calories in this book were rounded to the nearest 5, and all other amounts were rounded to the nearest .5 of a gram.

Net carbs are the carbs believed to digest and have an impact on your body. They were calculated by subtracting the grams of fiber from the total carbohydrates.

Though we have provided this nutritional information, our family has always made it a point to not count each and every gram of carbohydrates or calories. It is our belief that if you stock your home full of naturally low-carb foods, you'll be eating well enough to see results.

## About Sugar Substitutes

Many of the recipes in this book call for sugar substitute. Your choice of sugar substitute is totally up to you, as long as it meets two requirements:

1. It measures the same as real sugar, cup for cup.
2. It is heat-stable and won't lose its sweetness as it cooks. Aspartame (Equal) is not heat-stable.

Our family uses Splenda, but there are a ton of options available today—including all-natural options. These include stevia, monk-fruit, and erythritol.

# Pantry List

This is a list of the most commonly used pantry ingredients in this book. Keep many of these on hand for shorter shopping lists in the future.

### PANTRY
- Almond flour
- Cocoa powder
- Dijon mustard
- Garlic, minced
- Onions, red
- Onions, yellow
- Soy sauce
- Stock, chicken
- Stock, beef
- Stock, vegetable
- Sugar substitute
- Worcestershire sauce

### SPICE CABINET
- Bay leaves
- Black pepper
- Cayenne pepper
- Chili powder
- Chipotle chili powder
- Cinnamon, ground
- Crushed red pepper flakes
- Cumin, ground
- Diced tomatoes, petite
- Five-spice powder
- Garam masala
- Garlic powder
- Italian seasoning
- Nonstick cooking spray
- Oil, olive
- Oil, sesame
- Oil, vegetable
- Onion powder
- Oregano
- Paprika
- Salt
- Sherry cooking wine
- Smoked paprika
- Thyme
- Tomato paste
- Vanilla extract
- Vinegar, balsamic
- Vinegar, cider
- Vinegar, rice wine
- Vinegar, white

### FRIDGE
- Basil, fresh
- Bell peppers
- Butter
- Cauliflower
- Cilantro
- Cream cheese
- Dill, fresh
- Eggs, large
- Heavy cream
- Lemons
- Limes
- Parmesan cheese
- Parsley
- Rosemary, fresh
- Sage, fresh
- Thyme, fresh

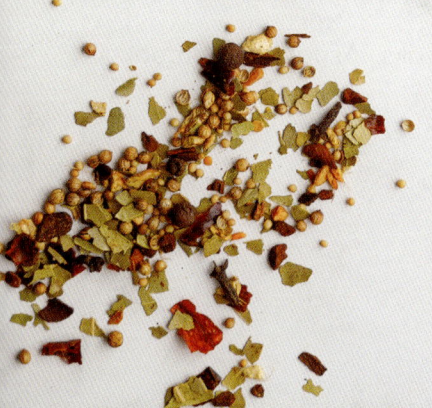

Instant Low Carb • 21

*Chapter 1*

# Breakfast

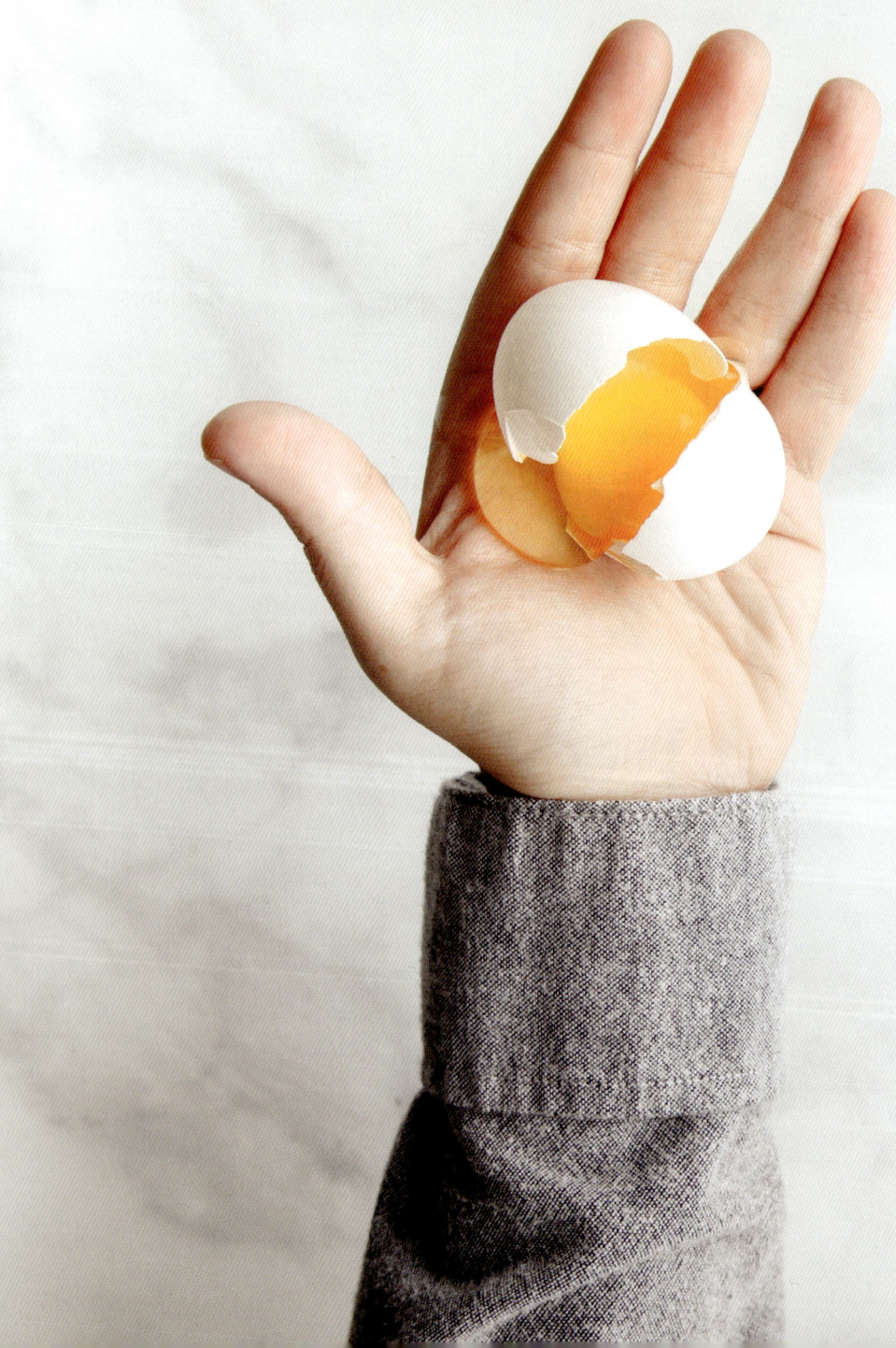

## recipes in this chapter...

**Mushroom Swiss Coddled Eggs**, 25
**Denver Egg Bites**, 27
**Chicken Sausage and Gouda Frittata**, 28
**Sausage and Sweet Potato Hash**, 29
**Southwestern Shirred Eggs**, 31
**Spinach and Goat Cheese Egg Cups**, 32
**Quiche Lorraine**, 33
**Steak and Eggplant Hash**, 35
**Pepperoni Pizza Egg Bites**, 36
**Perfect Poached Eggs**, 37
**Broccoli Cheese Quiche**, 39
**Blueberry Muffin Cups**, 41

*We thought it would be fun to write secret messages around the edge of this plate. Sorry the type is so small, but if it were any larger, it wouldn't be a secret message anymore.*

**Breakfast**

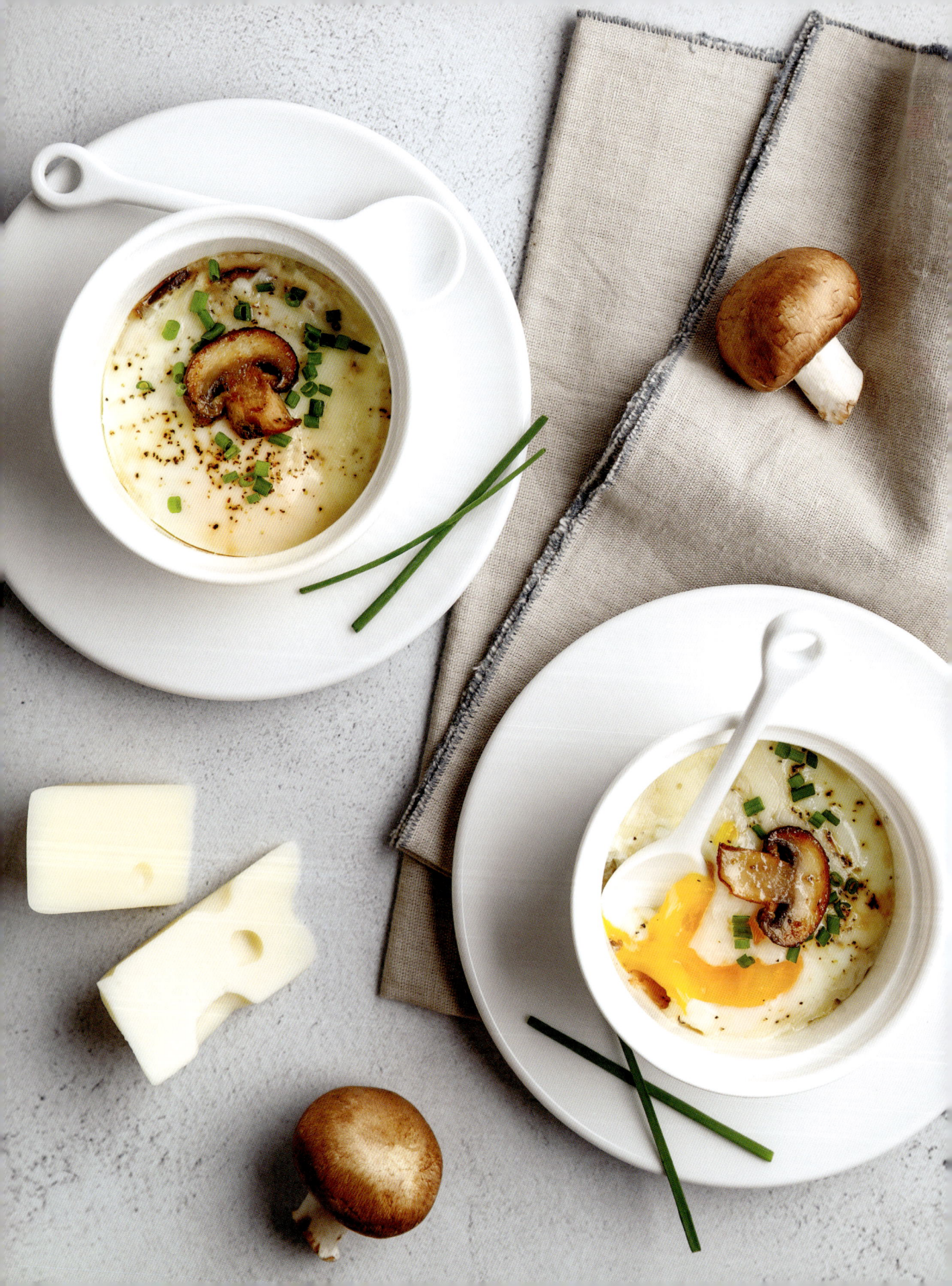

Prep Time: 10 min  |  High Pressure: 1 min  |  Natural Release: 2 min  |  Serves: 4

# Mushroom Swiss Coddled Eggs

We love cooking eggs in the Instant Pot, but it can be a bit tricky to get a nice, soft yolk. We've found that times can vary each time you make them, depending on the exact size of the egg, size and thickness of the ramekins, or how much water is added to the water bath. One minute at high pressure with 2 minutes of natural release has been the most foolproof for us as it errs on the side of undercooking, rather than overcooking, as you can always put the lid back on to continue steaming these using just the residual heat left in the cooker.

## Ingredients

Nonstick cooking spray
1 tablespoon butter
6 baby bella mushrooms, sliced
¼ teaspoon salt
¼ teaspoon pepper
⅛ teaspoon garlic powder
¼ cup shredded Swiss cheese
4 large eggs
1 tablespoon chopped chives

## Special Equipment

4 ramekins
Steam rack

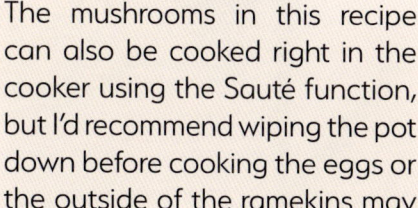

**Instant Tips**

The mushrooms in this recipe can also be cooked right in the cooker using the Sauté function, but I'd recommend wiping the pot down before cooking the eggs or the outside of the ramekins may get greasy.

1. Pour 1 cup of water into the Instant Pot. Spray 4 ramekins with nonstick cooking spray.

2. Heat butter in a small skillet over medium-high heat. Add mushrooms, salt, pepper, and garlic powder to the skillet and sauté just until mushrooms begin to brown.

3. Spoon an equal amount of the mushrooms into each ramekin. Top mushrooms in each with ⅛ of the shredded Swiss cheese (a large pinch).

4. Crack a whole egg over top of the mushrooms in each ramekin, then season lightly with salt and pepper. Top with an equal amount of the remaining Swiss cheese.

5. Cover each ramekin tightly with aluminum foil, then arrange all 4 on the steam rack. Carefully lower into the water bath in the Instant Pot.

6. Lock lid in place and seal pressure release vent. Set cooker to HIGH pressure for 1 minute.

7. Let pressure release naturally for just 2 minutes before opening vent to release any remaining pressure.

8. Uncover immediately and check eggs for doneness. If egg whites are not firm, place lid back on the cooker (with all settings off) for 1 minute, just to let the residual heat finish the cooking. Serve in the ramekins, topped with chopped chives.

*Breakfast*

---

Calories: 125  |  Fat: 10g  |  Protein: 8.5g  |  Total Carbs: 1g  -  Fiber: 0g  =  Net Carbs: 1g

Instant Low Carb • 25

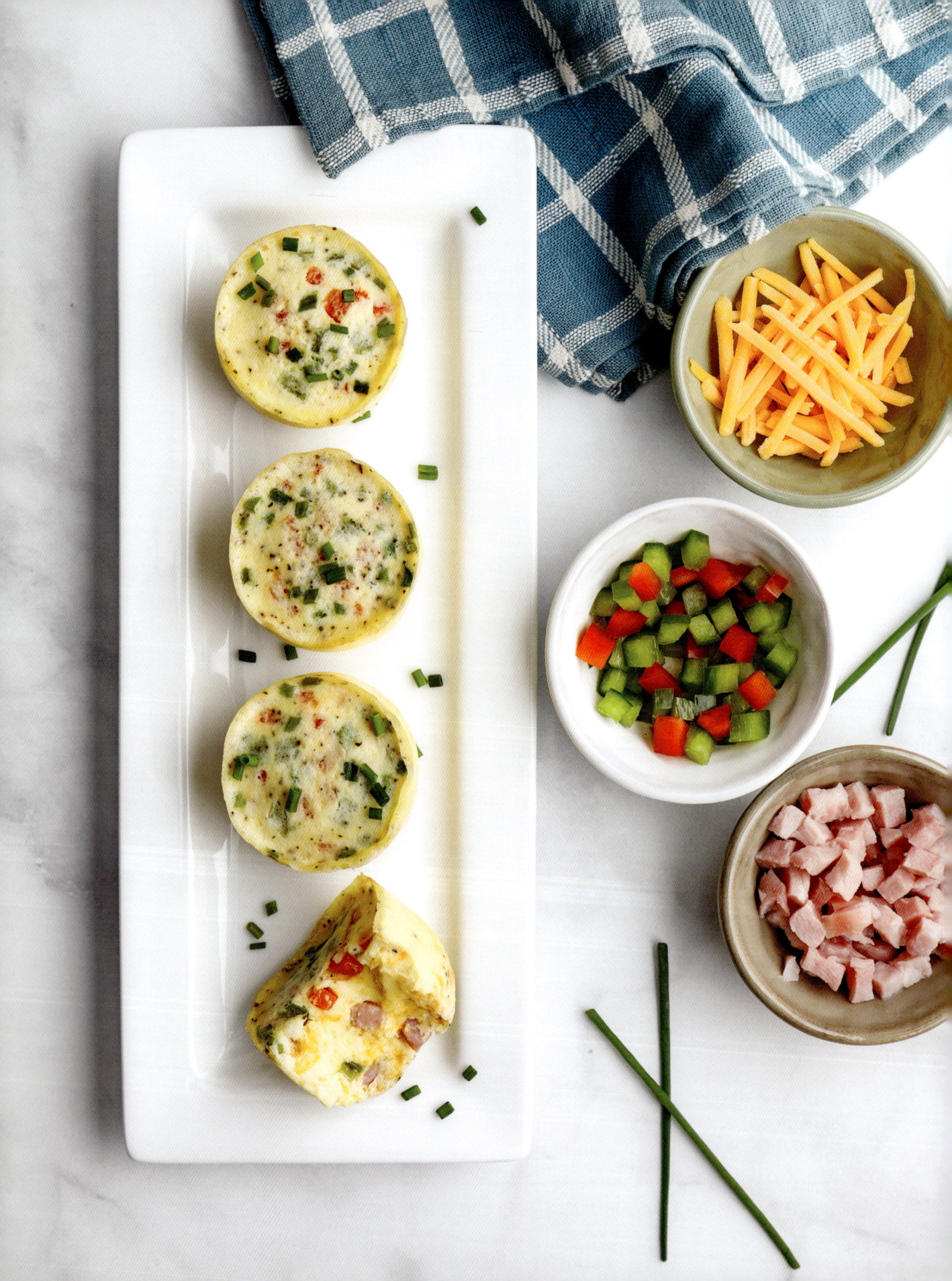

**Prep Time: 10 min | High Pressure: 10 min | Natural Release: 5 min | Makes: 7**

# Denver Egg Bites

We've been making scrambled egg muffins (using traditional muffin pans) for as long as we can remember, so we were happy when "Egg Bites" became such a hot new food. It meant that we could finally get a silicone mold that fit into our Instant Pot! For the lightest and fluffiest bites, we use a blender to whip up the batter of eggs and cheese before pouring over the ham and bell pepper that you'll always find in a classic Denver Omelet.

## Ingredients

Nonstick cooking spray
¼ cup diced ham
¼ cup finely diced bell pepper, any color
1 tablespoon chopped chives
4 large eggs
½ cup shredded sharp Cheddar cheese
¼ cup heavy cream
¼ teaspoon salt
¼ teaspoon pepper

### Special Equipment
Egg bites mold
Steam rack

1. Pour 1 cup of water into the Instant Pot. Spray egg bites mold with nonstick cooking spray.

2. Evenly distribute the ham, bell pepper, and chives between the 7 cups of the egg bites mold.

3. In a blender or food processor, blend the eggs, Cheddar cheese, heavy cream, salt, and pepper, until mostly smooth.

4. Pour the egg mixture over top of the ingredients in each cup of the egg bites mold. For best results, use a fork to disperse ingredients evenly throughout each egg bite.

5. Cover egg bites mold with aluminum foil before placing on steam rack. Carefully lower into the water bath in the Instant Pot.

6. Lock lid in place and seal pressure release vent. Set cooker to HIGH pressure for 10 minutes.

7. Let pressure release naturally for 5 minutes before opening vent to release any remaining pressure.

8. Let cool 2 minutes before popping egg bites out of the mold to serve.

*Breakfast*

**Instant Tips**

Stir the egg batter as you pour it into the molds to ensure the cheese is evenly added to each bite, as it likes to sink to the bottom of the blender.

---

**Calories: 115 | Fat: 9g | Protein: 6.5g | Total Carbs: 1g - Fiber: 0g = Net Carbs: 1g**

Prep Time: 10 min | High Pressure: 25 min | Natural Release: 10 min | Serves: 6

# Chicken Sausage and Gouda Frittata

This egg white frittata is light but still fulfilling and packed with the smoky flavors of chicken sausage and gouda cheese. Any flavor of smoked chicken sausage will work but be sure to check the package for any added sugars. Andouille sausage can also be used.

## Ingredients

Nonstick cooking spray

4 links smoked chicken sausage, chopped

1 cup shredded smoked gouda cheese

¼ cup diced red bell pepper

8 large egg whites

½ cup heavy cream

¼ teaspoon onion powder

½ teaspoon salt

¼ teaspoon pepper

## Special Equipment

7-inch springform pan

Steam rack

1. Pour 1 cup of water into the Instant Pot. Spray a 7-inch springform pan with nonstick cooking spray.
2. Add sausage, gouda cheese, and bell pepper to the prepared pan.
3. In a mixing bowl, whisk together egg whites, heavy cream, onion powder, salt, and pepper.
4. Pour the egg mixture over top of the ingredients in the prepared pan and stir to evenly disperse the sausage and cheese.
5. Tightly wrap the bottom and top of the pan to ensure it is watertight before placing on steam rack. Carefully lower into the water bath in the Instant Pot.
6. Lock lid in place and seal pressure release vent. Set cooker to HIGH pressure for 25 minutes.
7. Let pressure release naturally for 10 minutes before opening vent to release any remaining pressure.
8. Let cool 5 minutes before unlocking springform pan, slicing, and serving.

**Instant Tips**

We like to add a seeded and finely diced jalapeño to this as well for even more color and flavor, but it cooks up pretty spicy as the peppers aren't sautéed before adding to the frittata.

Calories: 235 | Fat: 17g | Protein: 18g | Total Carbs: 3g - Fiber: 0g = Net Carbs: 3g

Prep Time: 10 min | High Pressure: 3 min | Quick Release | Serves: 6

# Sausage and Sweet Potato Hash

Crumbled breakfast sausage and chopped sweet potato are the stars of this savory hash with just a hint of sweetness. It's great when topped with eggs or even served as a side dish (in place of stuffing) around the holidays.

## Ingredients

2 tablespoons butter, divided

1 pound ground breakfast sausage

1 large sweet potato, chopped large

½ cup diced yellow onion

½ cup diced yellow bell pepper

2 teaspoons sugar substitute

¼ teaspoon ground cinnamon

¼ teaspoon onion powder

¼ teaspoon salt

¼ teaspoon pepper

½ cup chicken stock

3 leaves sage, chopped

1. Heat 1 tablespoon of the butter in the Instant Pot set to SAUTÉ.

2. Once butter is sizzling, add sausage and brown well, crumbling as it cooks. Drain excess grease and remove sausage from cooker, setting aside.

3. Add the remaining tablespoon of butter, sweet potato, onion, bell pepper, sugar substitute, cinnamon, onion powder, salt, and pepper to the cooker and sauté until sweet potato begins to brown.

4. Add the chicken stock to the cooker, lock lid in place, and seal pressure release vent. Set cooker to HIGH pressure for 3 minutes.

5. Carefully open vent to quickly release the pressure. For best texture, drain liquid from cooker.

6. Return the sausage to the vegetables in the cooker and add sage, folding everything together before serving.

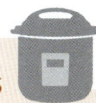

### Instant Tips

There are a couple of extra steps in this recipe that aren't necessary, but we find they make for better texture and flavor. The sausage does not have to be removed from the cooker before cooking potatoes under pressure and the liquid does not need to be drained after cooking if you serve using a slotted spoon.

Calories: 325 | Fat: 25g | Protein: 15.5g | Total Carbs: 8g - Fiber: 1.5g = Net Carbs: 6.5g

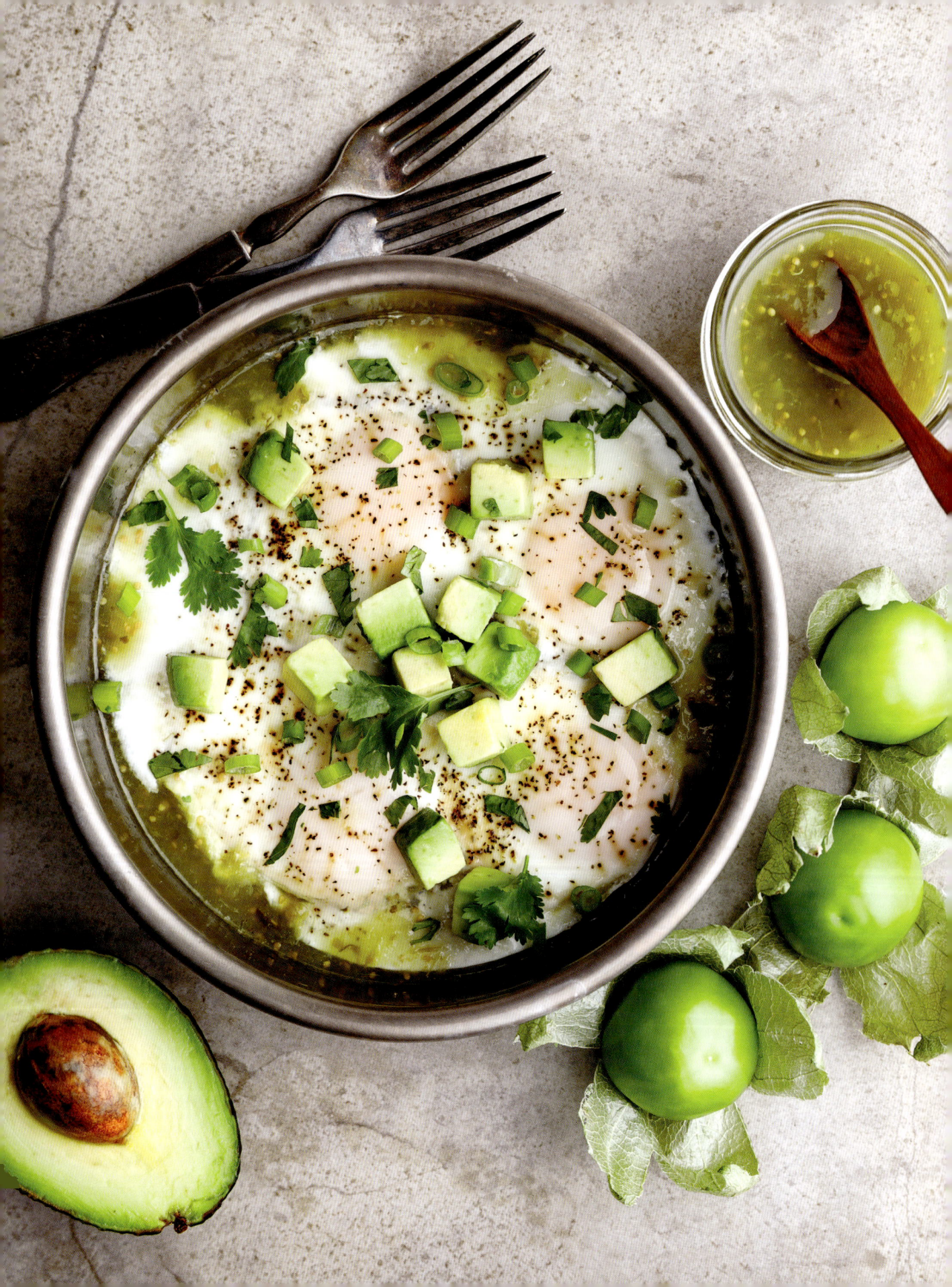

Prep Time: 10 min | High Pressure: 3 min | Quick Release | Serves: 2

# Southwestern Shirred Eggs

A fancy name for baked eggs, these "Shirred Eggs" are cooked in a bed of tomatillo salsa verde and topped with avocado, scallions, and cilantro. It's a beautiful presentation of fresh and green ingredients that makes for a deliciously different breakfast.

## Ingredients

Nonstick cooking spray

1/3 cup salsa verde (see tip)

4 large eggs

Salt and pepper

1/2 avocado, chopped

2 scallions, chopped

2 tablespoons chopped cilantro

## Special Equipment

7-inch cake pan

Steam rack

1. Pour 1 cup of water into the Instant Pot. Spray a 7-inch cake pan with nonstick cooking spray.
2. Spread salsa over the bottom of the cake pan and crack the 4 eggs over top.
3. Season lightly with salt and pepper before covering with aluminum foil.
4. Lock lid in place and seal pressure release vent. Set cooker to HIGH pressure for 3 minutes.
5. Quickly release the pressure by carefully opening the vent to let out all steam.
6. Uncover eggs and check whites for doneness. If whites are not firm, leave uncovered and loosely place the lid back on the Instant Pot for 1–2 minutes (with all settings off) to let the residual heat steam the tops of the eggs.
7. Top with avocado, scallions, and cilantro before serving.

*Breakfast*

### Instant Tips

Look for a brand of salsa verde without any added sugar. We use Herdez brand, as it is the most widely available and only has a few ingredients which are all low-carb friendly.

Calories: 240 | Fat: 15.5g | Protein: 14g | Total Carbs: 8g - Fiber: 3g = Net Carbs: 5g

Instant Low Carb • 31

Prep Time: 10 min | High Pressure: 1 min | Natural Release: 3 min | Serves: 4

# Spinach and Goat Cheese Egg Cups

These egg cups are made in ceramic ramekins with whole eggs over top a bed of chopped spinach, garlic, and roasted red bell peppers. The cups are topped off with creamy herbed goat cheese for a farm fresh-flavor through and through.

## Ingredients

Nonstick cooking spray

1/3 cup frozen chopped spinach, thawed and drained

2 tablespoons diced roasted red pepper

1 teaspoon minced garlic

1/4 teaspoon salt

1/4 teaspoon pepper

4 large eggs

2 ounces creamy herbed goat cheese

## Special Equipment

4 ramekins

Steam rack

1. Pour 1 cup of water into the Instant Pot. Spray 4 ramekins with nonstick cooking spray.
2. In a mixing bowl, fold together spinach, roasted red pepper, garlic, salt, and pepper.
3. Spoon an equal amount of the spinach mixture into each ramekin.
4. Crack a whole egg over top of the spinach in each ramekin, then season lightly with salt and pepper. Top with an equal amount of the herbed goat cheese.
5. Cover each ramekin tightly with aluminum foil, then arrange all 4 on the steam rack. Carefully lower into the water bath in the Instant Pot.
6. Lock lid in place and seal pressure release vent. Set cooker to HIGH pressure for 1 minute.
7. Let pressure release naturally for 3 minutes before opening vent to release any remaining pressure.
8. Uncover immediately and check eggs for doneness. If egg whites are not firm, place lid back on the cooker (with all settings off) for 1 minute, just to let the residual heat finish the cooking. Serve directly in the ramekins.

### Instant Tips

Herbed goat cheese is often sold in small cylinders in the imported/fancy cheese section. Regular goat cheese can be substituted in its place, if needed.

Calories: 140 | Fat: 10g | Protein: 10.5g | Total Carbs: 1.5g - Fiber: 0g = Net Carbs: 1.5g

Prep Time: 10 min | High Pressure: 30 min | Natural Release: 5 min | Serves: 6

# Quiche Lorraine

This classic quiche is made crustless and cooked under pressure for a rich and creamy texture that's hard to achieve outside of the Instant Pot. We love using fresh thyme leaves in this for a bright and clean flavor, but ½ teaspoon of dried can be used in a pinch.

## Ingredients

Nonstick cooking spray
8 strips cooked bacon, crumbled
1 ½ cups shredded Swiss cheese
3 tablespoons minced shallot
7 large eggs
⅔ cup heavy cream
2 teaspoons fresh thyme leaves
½ teaspoon salt
¼ teaspoon pepper
⅛ teaspoon onion powder
Pinch ground nutmeg

## Special Equipment

7-inch springform pan
Steam rack

1. Pour 1 cup of water into the Instant Pot. Spray a 7-inch springform pan with nonstick cooking spray.
2. Add crumbled bacon, Swiss cheese, and shallot to the prepared pan.
3. In a mixing bowl, whisk together eggs, heavy cream, thyme, salt, pepper, onion powder, and nutmeg.
4. Pour the egg mixture over top of the ingredients in the prepared pan and stir to evenly disperse the bacon and cheese.
5. Tightly wrap the bottom and top of the pan to ensure it is watertight before placing on steam rack. Carefully lower into the water bath in the Instant Pot.
6. Lock lid in place and seal pressure release vent. Set cooker to HIGH pressure for 30 minutes.
7. Let pressure release naturally for 5 minutes before opening vent to release any remaining pressure.
8. Let cool 5 minutes before unlocking springform pan, slicing, and serving warm. Cover and refrigerate to serve chilled. For a better presentation, sprinkle additional shredded Swiss cheese over top as soon as you remove it from the cooker.

**Instant Tips**

For a bit of spice, add 1 teaspoon of hot sauce to the egg mixture as you whisk it together.

Calories: 370 | Fat: 41.5g | Protein: 20g | Total Carbs: 3.5g - Fiber: 0g = Net Carbs: 3.5g

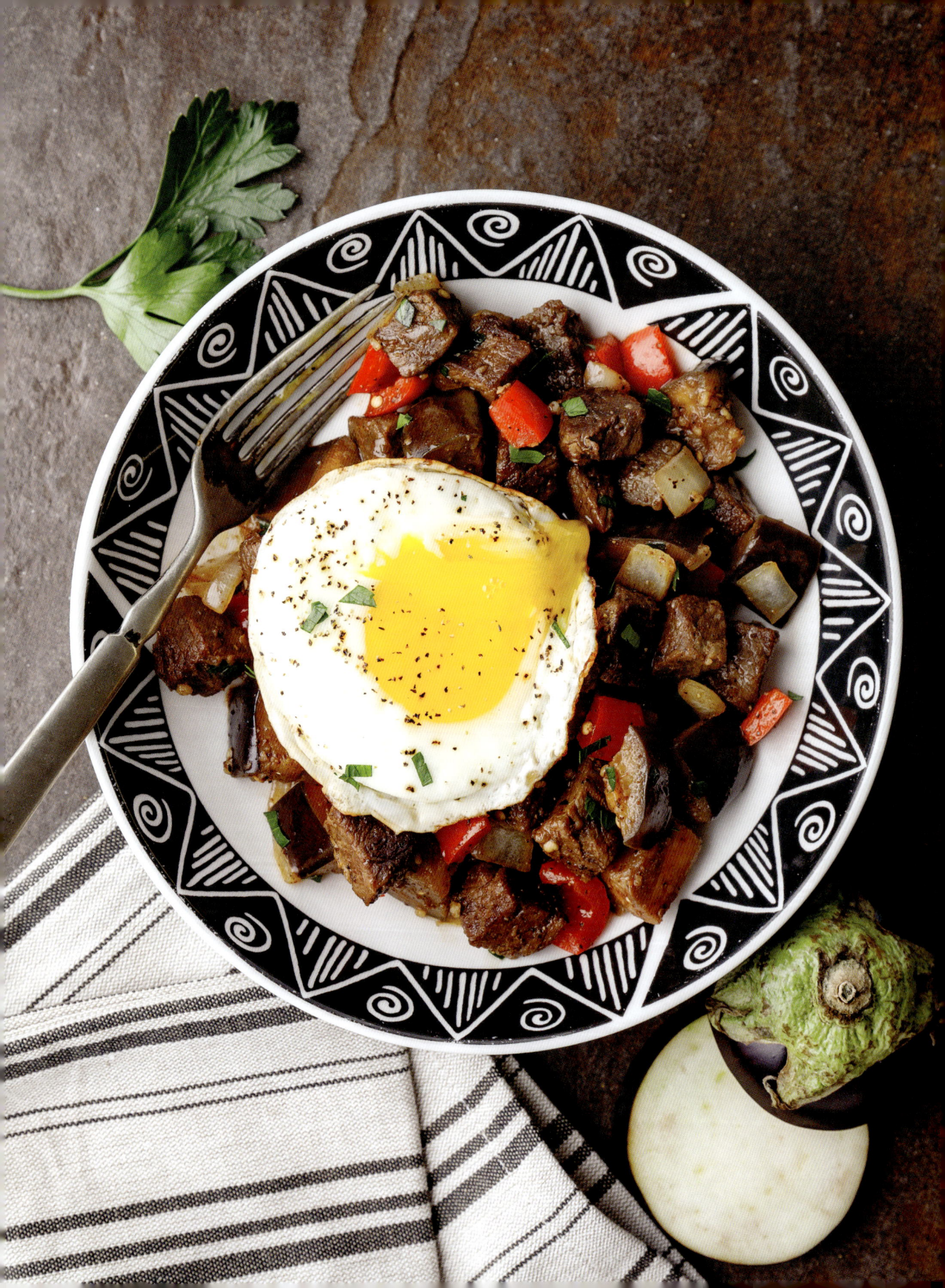

**Prep Time:** 10 min  |  **High Pressure:** 20 min  |  **Natural Release:** 5 min  |  **Serves:** 4

# Steak and Eggplant Hash

Sirloin steak is chopped and cooked until it is as tender as pot roast before adding to this breakfast hash with eggplant, onion, and bell pepper. It's a lot more convenient than preparing corned beef hash, as corned beef can get pricey and isn't sold in small enough packages for breakfast.

## Ingredients

- 1 pound sirloin steak, cut into ¾-inch cubes
- Salt and pepper
- 1 cup beef stock
- 2 tablespoons vegetable oil
- 1 tablespoon butter
- 1 small eggplant, cut into ¾-inch cubes
- ½ cup diced yellow onion
- ½ cup diced red bell pepper
- 2 teaspoons minced garlic
- ½ teaspoon chili powder
- ¼ teaspoon onion powder
- 1 tablespoon chopped parsley

1. Generously season steak with salt and pepper before transferring to the Instant Pot.
2. Add the beef stock to the cooker, lock lid in place, and seal pressure release vent. Set cooker to HIGH pressure for 20 minutes.
3. Let pressure release naturally for 5 minutes before opening vent to release any remaining pressure. Drain all liquid.
4. Set cooker to SAUTÉ and add all remaining ingredients except parsley.
5. Sauté for 10 minutes or until eggplant is tender and steak has begun to brown.
6. Stir in chopped parsley before serving.

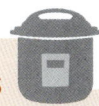

**Instant Tips**

You can also cook the eggplant, onions, and peppers in a large skillet on the stove over medium-high heat as the steak is cooking in the Instant Pot. Then add the cooked steak to the skillet for just 3 or 4 minutes of sautéing before serving.

**Calories:** 320  |  **Fat:** 17g  |  **Protein:** 35.5g  |  **Total Carbs:** 5.5g  -  **Fiber:** 2g  =  **Net Carbs:** 3.5g

Prep Time: 10 min | High Pressure: 10 min | Natural Release: 5 min | Makes: 7

# Pepperoni Pizza Egg Bites

You can have pizza for breakfast with these savory egg bites. We like to use turkey pepperoni in place of regular pepperoni, as the grease of regular pepperoni doesn't mix well with the eggs. For even fresher flavors, sprinkle a tablespoon of chopped fresh basil evenly between each bite before adding the egg batter, then serve topped with diced fresh tomato or a side of sugar-free tomato sauce for dipping.

*Breakfast*

## Ingredients

Nonstick cooking spray

1/3 cup diced turkey pepperoni

2 tablespoons finely diced green bell pepper

4 large eggs

1/2 cup shredded mozzarella cheese

1/4 cup heavy cream

1/4 teaspoon salt

1/4 teaspoon pepper

1/8 teaspoon garlic powder

1/2 teaspoon Italian seasoning

## Special Equipment

Egg bites mold

Steam rack

1. Pour 1 cup of water into the Instant Pot. Spray egg bites mold with nonstick cooking spray.

2. Evenly distribute the pepperoni and bell pepper between the 7 cups of the egg bites mold.

3. In a blender or food processor, blend the eggs, mozzarella cheese, heavy cream, salt, pepper, and garlic powder until mostly smooth. Stir in Italian seasoning after blending.

4. Pour the egg mixture over top of the ingredients in each cup of the egg bites mold. For best results, use a fork to disperse ingredients evenly throughout each egg bite.

5. Cover egg bites mold with aluminum foil before placing on steam rack. Carefully lower into the water bath in the Instant Pot.

6. Lock lid in place and seal pressure release vent. Set cooker to HIGH pressure for 10 minutes.

7. Let pressure release naturally for 5 minutes before opening vent to release any remaining pressure.

8. Let cool 2 minutes before popping egg bites out of the mold to serve.

**Instant Tips**

Stir the egg batter as you pour it into the molds to ensure the cheese is evenly added to each bite, as it likes to sink to the bottom of the blender.

Calories: 125 | Fat: 8.5g | Protein: 8.5g | Total Carbs: 3g - Fiber: 0.5g = Net Carbs: 2.5g

**Prep Time: 2 min | High Pressure: 4 min | Quick Release | Makes: 1–7**

# Perfect Poached Eggs

Poaching eggs in the Instant Pot is more about convenience than speed, especially when you are multitasking in the kitchen. We've found that we get the most consistent results by only partially cooking the eggs under pressure, then switching to the SAUTÉ setting to steam for the final minute or two under a glass lid. There are too many variables (desired amount of eggs being cooked, the age of the eggs, exact size of the eggs, temperature of steaming water at start, varying thickness between different brands of silicone egg molds) to recommend cooking the eggs under pressure alone. Thankfully, with the Instant Pot, you can simply hit a switch to change cook settings in an instant.

## Ingredients

Nonstick cooking spray
1–7 large eggs

## Special Equipment

Egg bites mold
Steam rack
Glass lid

1. Pour 1 cup of water into the Instant Pot. Spray egg bites mold with nonstick cooking spray.

2. Crack one egg into each of the desired number of egg bites cups.

3. Place egg bites mold on steam rack and carefully lower into the water bath in the Instant Pot. Do NOT cover egg bites mold with aluminum foil.

4. Lock lid in place and seal pressure release vent. Set cooker to HIGH pressure for 4 minutes.

5. Open vent to quickly release the pressure. Use the back of a spoon to check egg whites for doneness and yolks for desired firmness. They will likely be slightly undercooked.

6. Set cooker to SAUTÉ and cover pot with glass lid. Let cook, checking at least every minute, until whites have set and yolks are to your desired doneness.

7. Use a spoon to release eggs from the mold. Unlike other recipes made in the egg bites mold, inverting the mold and popping the eggs out is not recommended, as the yolks may break.

> **Instant Tips**
> We like to add a tablespoon or two of butter to one of the empty egg bites cups before the sauté step to melt it for drizzling over the finished poached eggs.

**Calories: 70 | Fat: 5g | Protein: 6g | Total Carbs: 0g - Fiber: 0g = Net Carbs: 0g**

Instant Low Carb • 37

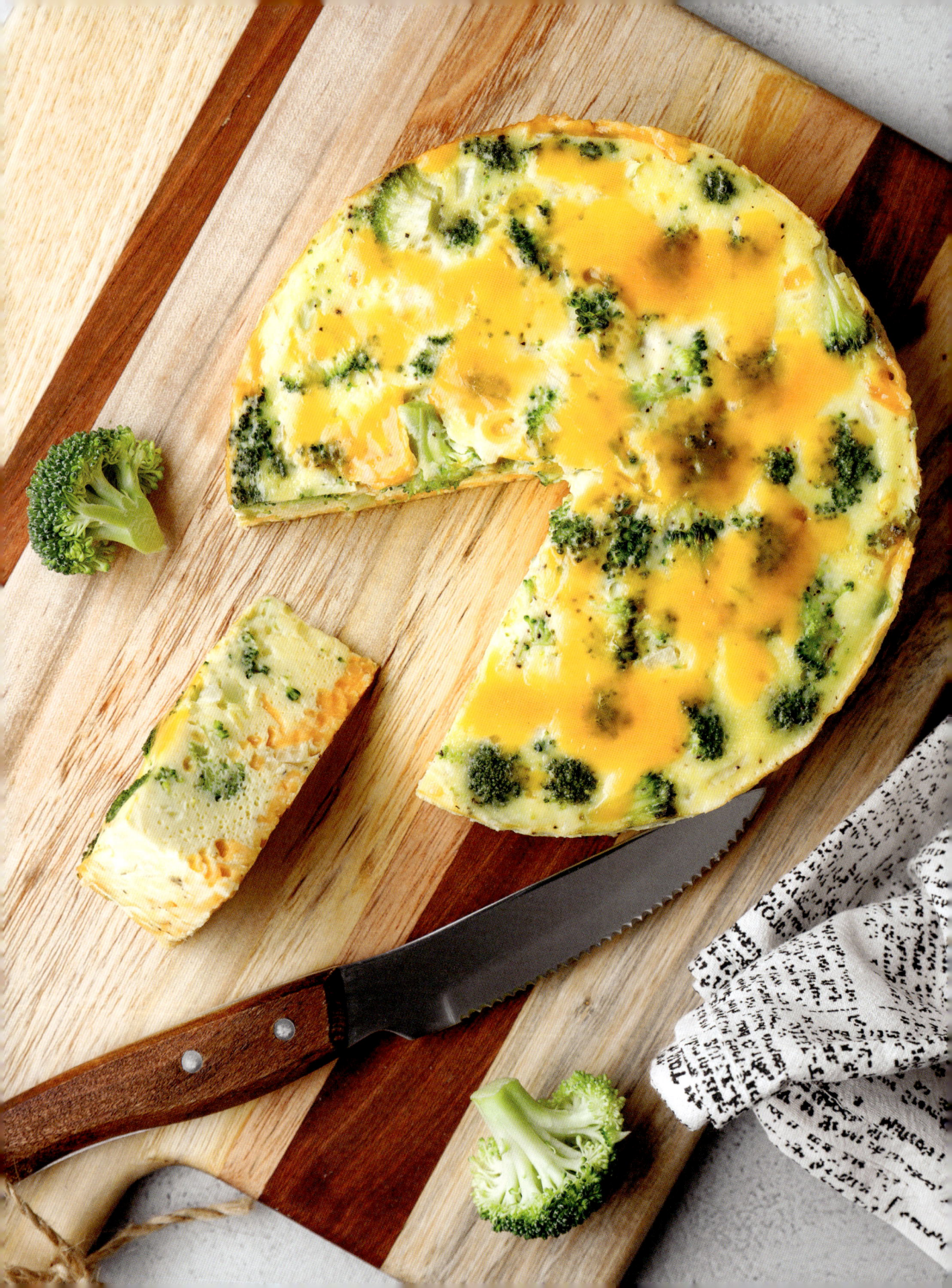

Prep Time: 10 min | High Pressure: 25 min | Natural Release: 10 min | Serves: 6

# Broccoli Cheese Quiche

This crustless quiche makes up for its smaller diameter (to fit into the Instant Pot) with an impressive height. The combination of fresh broccoli, Cheddar cheese, and a touch of yellow onion used in the filling is not only a classic but family-friendly as well.

## Ingredients

Nonstick cooking spray

1 cup chopped broccoli florets

1 cup shredded sharp Cheddar cheese

2 tablespoons minced yellow onion

6 large eggs

½ cup heavy cream

½ teaspoon salt

¼ teaspoon pepper

⅛ teaspoon garlic powder

Pinch ground nutmeg

## Special Equipment

7-inch springform pan

Steam rack

1. Pour 1 cup of water into the Instant Pot. Spray a 7-inch springform pan with nonstick cooking spray.
2. Add broccoli, Cheddar cheese, and onion to the prepared pan.
3. In a mixing bowl, whisk together eggs, heavy cream, salt, pepper, garlic powder, and nutmeg.
4. Pour the egg mixture over top of the ingredients in the prepared pan and stir to evenly disperse the broccoli and cheese.
5. Tightly wrap the bottom and top of the pan to ensure it is watertight before placing on steam rack. Carefully lower into the water bath in the Instant Pot.
6. Lock lid in place and seal pressure release vent. Set cooker to HIGH pressure for 25 minutes.
7. Let pressure release naturally for 10 minutes before opening vent to release any remaining pressure.
8. Let cool 5 minutes before unlocking springform pan, slicing, and serving warm. Cover and refrigerate to serve chilled. For a better presentation, sprinkle additional shredded Cheddar cheese over top as soon as you remove it from the cooker.

**Breakfast**

### Instant Tips

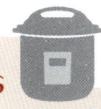

There's no need to precook or use frozen broccoli in this recipe, as fresh cooks up perfectly right inside the quiche.

Calories: 225 | Fat: 18.5g | Protein: 12g | Total Carbs: 3g - Fiber: 0.5g = Net Carbs: 2.5g

Instant Low Carb • 39

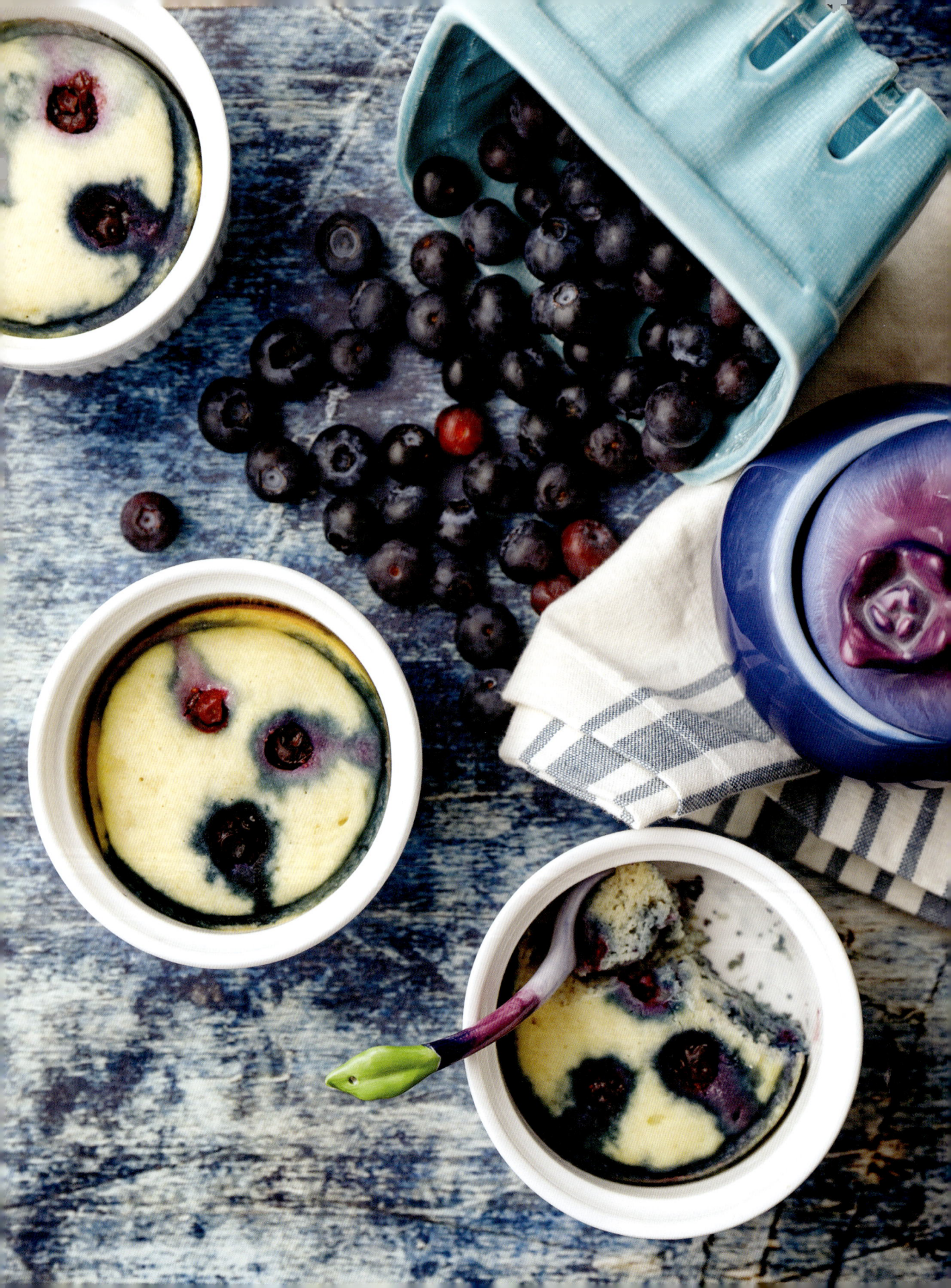

Prep Time: 10 min | High Pressure: 10 min | Natural Release: 5 min | Serves: 4

# Blueberry Muffin Cups

These muffin cups cook up soft and pillow-y under pressure, making for an easy breakfast served in a unique and interesting way. Just like traditional muffins, these are even better when served warm with a small pat of butter over top.

## Ingredients

Nonstick cooking spray
3/4 cup almond flour
1/3 cup + 1 tablespoon sugar substitute
1 teaspoon baking powder
1 large egg
2 large egg whites
2 tablespoons butter, melted
2 tablespoons water
1 teaspoon vanilla extract
1/3 cup blueberries

## Special Equipment

4 ramekins
Steam rack

1. Pour 1 cup of water into the Instant Pot. Spray 4 ramekins with nonstick cooking spray.

2. In a mixing bowl, combine almond flour, both measures of sugar substitute, and baking powder.

3. In a separate mixing bowl, whisk together egg, egg whites, butter, water, and vanilla extract.

4. Fold the wet ingredients into the dry ingredients until a batter is formed. Gently fold blueberries into the batter.

5. Spoon an equal amount of the batter into each prepared ramekin. Tap each ramekin on the counter to even out the top of the batter.

6. Cover each ramekin tightly with aluminum foil, then arrange all 4 on the steam rack. Carefully lower into the water bath in the Instant Pot.

7. Lock lid in place and seal pressure release vent. Set cooker to HIGH pressure for 10 minutes.

8. Let pressure release naturally for 5 minutes before opening vent to release any remaining pressure. Serve warm or chilled, right out of the ramekins.

### Instant Tips

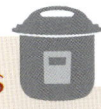

For a better presentation, lightly press 3 extra blueberries into the top of the batter in each ramekin before cooking. This ensures some blueberries will be visible in the final muffin cups.

Calories: 215 | Fat: 17.5g | Protein: 8g | Total Carbs: 9g - Fiber: 3g = Net Carbs: 6g

Chapter 2

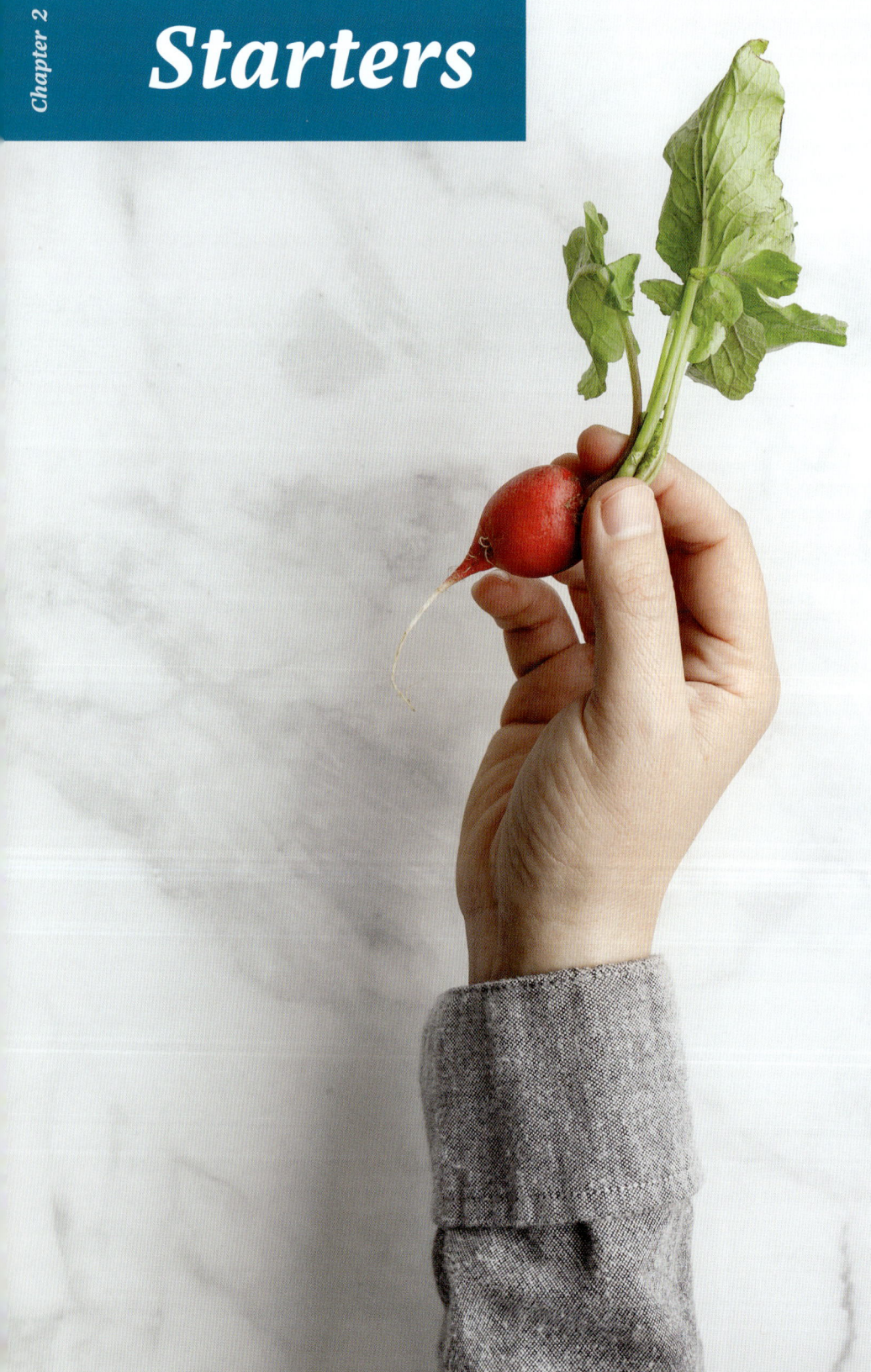

# *Starters*

## recipes in this chapter...

**Pickled Radishes, 45**

**Buffalo Wings, 47**

**Orange Ginger Edamame, 48**

**Whole Artichokes, 49**

**Greek Marinated Mushrooms, 51**

**Really Good Iced Tea, 53**

**Broccoli Cheese Dip, 54**

**Marinated Green Bean Antipasto, 55**

**Boiled Peanuts, 57**

**White "Bean" Dip with Pine Nuts, 59**

**Teriyaki Chicken Wings, 60**

**Instant Hard-Boiled Eggs, 61**

**Pimento-Cheese Deviled Eggs, 63**

*Secret Message #2: We didn't cook with many radishes until this past year but now we absolutely love them and love finding new ways to use them.*

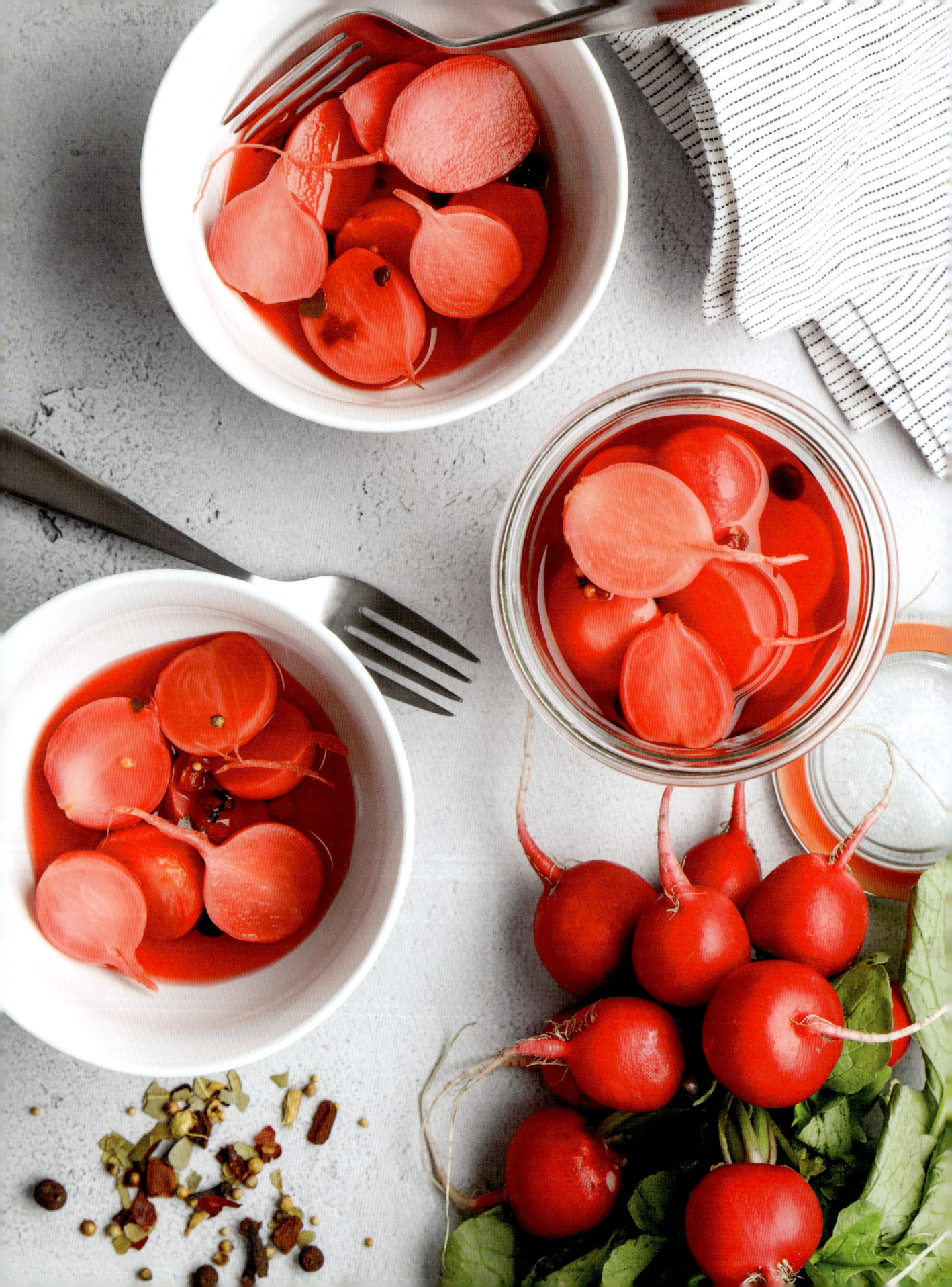

Prep Time: 10 min | High Pressure: 0 min | Quick Release | Serves: 6

# Pickled Radishes

We're officially going on record to say that we believe the radish to be the most overlooked and underused vegetable, and we're completely at a loss as to why. It truly is remarkable in that it takes on a completely different flavor when cooked, losing much of the spicy/bitter bite that raw radishes have and taking on a soft earthiness that is perfectly balanced during the pickling process.

## Ingredients

3/4 cup water
1/2 cup white vinegar
2 1/2 tablespoons sugar substitute
1 tablespoon pickling spice
1 1/2 teaspoons salt
2 cloves garlic
1 pound radishes, halved

## Special Equipment

Steam basket

1. Place all ingredients except radishes in the Instant Pot and stir to combine.
2. Place radishes in steam basket and lower into the cooker.
3. Lock lid in place and seal pressure release vent. Set cooker to HIGH pressure for 0 minutes.
4. Carefully open vent to quickly release the pressure.
5. Transfer radishes to a large food storage container or 2 jars.
6. Pour the liquid and all pickling ingredients from the cooker over the radishes.
7. Cover and refrigerate at least 4 hours before serving.

**Instant Tips**

These are also very good with a few chunks of fresh, peeled ginger added in the first step.

Calories: 15 | Fat: 0g | Protein: 0.5g | Total Carbs: 3g - Fiber: 1g = Net Carbs: 2g

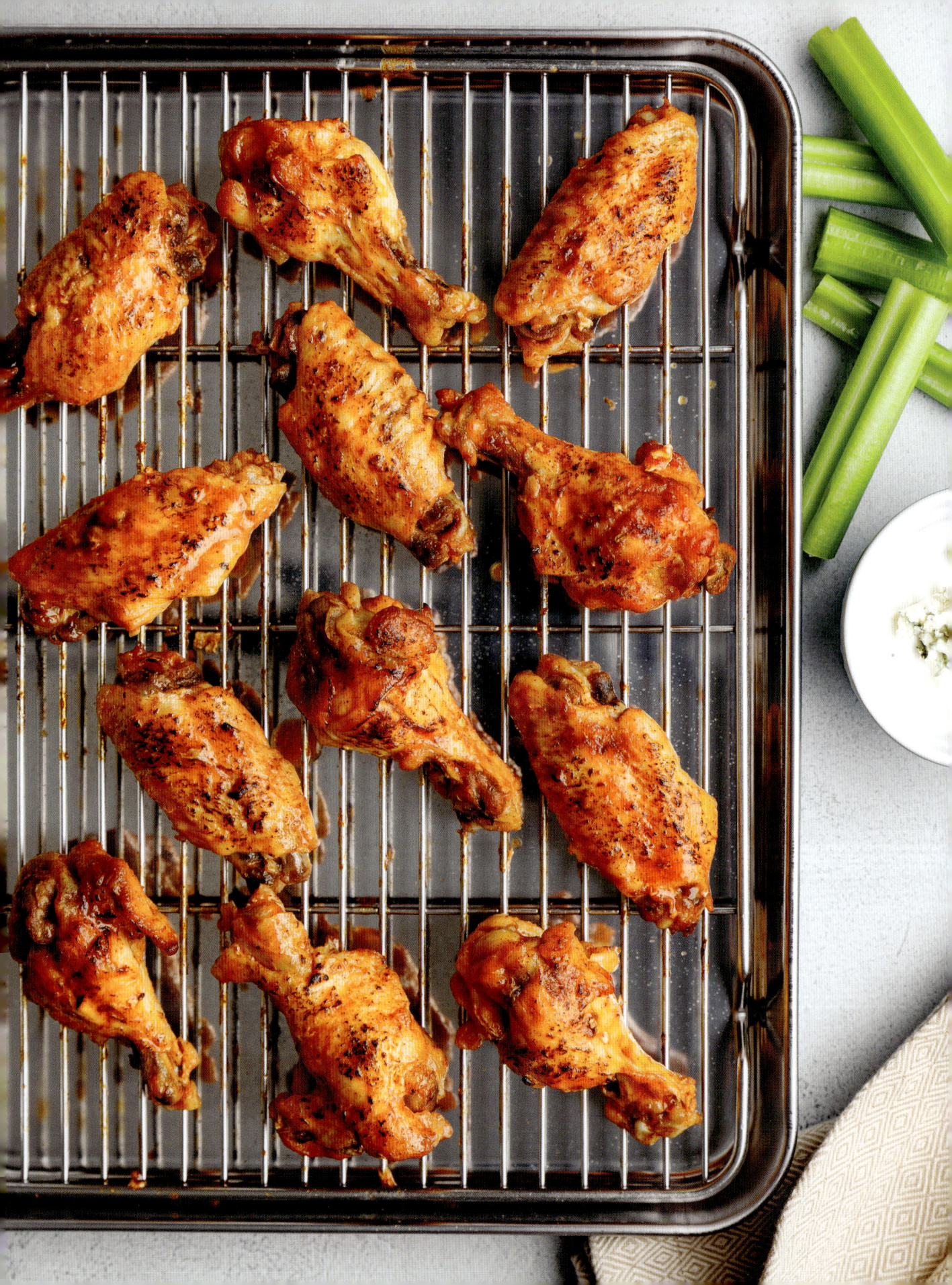

Prep Time: 5 min | High Pressure: 20 min | Quick Release | Serves: 6

# Buffalo Wings

While we are advocates of using fresh ingredients most of the time, using frozen here is easiest, as the wings and drums are already separated. To make a nice presentation and cool off the palate, serve this spicy chicken with blue cheese dressing and celery sticks.

## Ingredients

½ cup + 1 tablespoon buffalo sauce, divided

2 pounds frozen chicken wings

4 tablespoons butter, melted

## Special Equipment

Steam basket

1. Pour 1 cup water and 1 tablespoon of the buffalo sauce into the Instant Pot and place a steam basket over top.
2. Place chicken wings in the steam basket.
3. Lock lid in place and seal pressure release vent. Set cooker to HIGH pressure for 20 minutes.
4. Carefully open vent to quickly release the pressure.
5. Set oven to BROIL. In a large mixing bowl, combine remaining ½ cup buffalo sauce and butter to make the finished sauce.
6. Using tongs, transfer cooked wings to the mixing bowl and toss in the sauce to fully coat. Transfer to a broiler pan. Reserve mixing bowl of buffalo sauce.
7. Place wings under broiler for 4 minutes, just until chicken skin begins to crisp. Serve immediately. For even more flavor, flip wings and crisp the opposite side. Toss in the buffalo sauce a second time before serving.

### Instant Tips

We use Frank's Red Hot Buffalo Wings Sauce, which is pretty mild, to make these wings. If in doubt, you can also use any hot sauce labeled "Louisiana Hot Sauce" but it may be a bit spicy. If the sauce is too spicy for your taste, simply add more melted butter to cool down the heat.

Calories: 360 | Fat: 30g | Protein: 22.5g | Total Carbs: 0g - Fiber: 0g = Net Carbs: 0g

Prep Time: 5 min | High Pressure: 0 min | Quick Release | Serves: 4

# Orange Ginger Edamame

Edamame, or soybeans in the pod, are an often overlooked low-carb snack. It's like the Asian version of boiled peanuts—just as savory and addictive!

## Ingredients

1 (10-ounce) package frozen edamame in the pod

3 tablespoons soy sauce

½ cup vegetable stock

1 tablespoon sesame oil

1 tablespoon grated fresh ginger

2 teaspoons orange zest

2 teaspoons sugar substitute

1. Add all ingredients to the Instant Pot and toss to coat edamame.
2. Lock lid in place and seal pressure release vent. Set cooker to HIGH pressure for 0 minutes.
3. Carefully open vent to quickly release the pressure.
4. Serve the edamame drizzled with the cooking liquid.

### Instant Tips

Most frozen edamame is sold in 10-ounce packages, but some brands may vary. This recipe will work for up to 16 ounces without needing any adjustments.

Calories: 100 | Fat: 6g | Protein: 7g | Total Carbs: 6.5g - Fiber: 2.5g = Net Carbs: 4g

**Prep Time:** 10 min | **High Pressure:** 8 min | **Quick Release** | **Serves:** 3

# Whole Artichokes

It may be a new concept to some, but it isn't just the heart of an artichoke that is edible. In fact, there is quite a bit of meat on the leaves of these big bulbs. Boiling artichokes typically takes about 45 minutes on the stove, while cooking under pressure has them ready to eat in way less than half that time!

## Ingredients

3 medium artichokes
Juice of ½ lemon

## Special Equipment

Steam rack

1. Pour 1 cup of water into the Instant Pot and place a steam rack over top.
2. Use a chef's knife to trim most of the stem at the bottom of the artichokes. Then use one cutting motion to trim 1 inch from the entire top of each artichoke.
3. Arrange artichokes on steam rack stem sides down. Drizzle lemon juice over the top of each to prevent browning.
4. Lock lid in place and seal pressure release vent. Set cooker to HIGH pressure for 8 minutes.
5. Carefully open vent to quickly release the pressure.
6. To eat, pull the leaves from the artichoke one at a time and use your teeth to scrape the meat out of the bottom of the leaf. Discard tops of leaves. Once all leaves are gone, use a spoon to scrape away all of the fuzzy, inedible core (the "choke") of the artichoke, leaving only the tender heart.

### Instant Tips

Artichokes love a simple dipping sauce! Dip the leaves into melted butter with minced garlic or mayonnaise with a splash of lemon juice.

**Calories:** 60 | **Fat:** 0g | **Protein:** 4g | **Total Carbs:** 13g - **Fiber:** 7g = **Net Carbs:** 6g

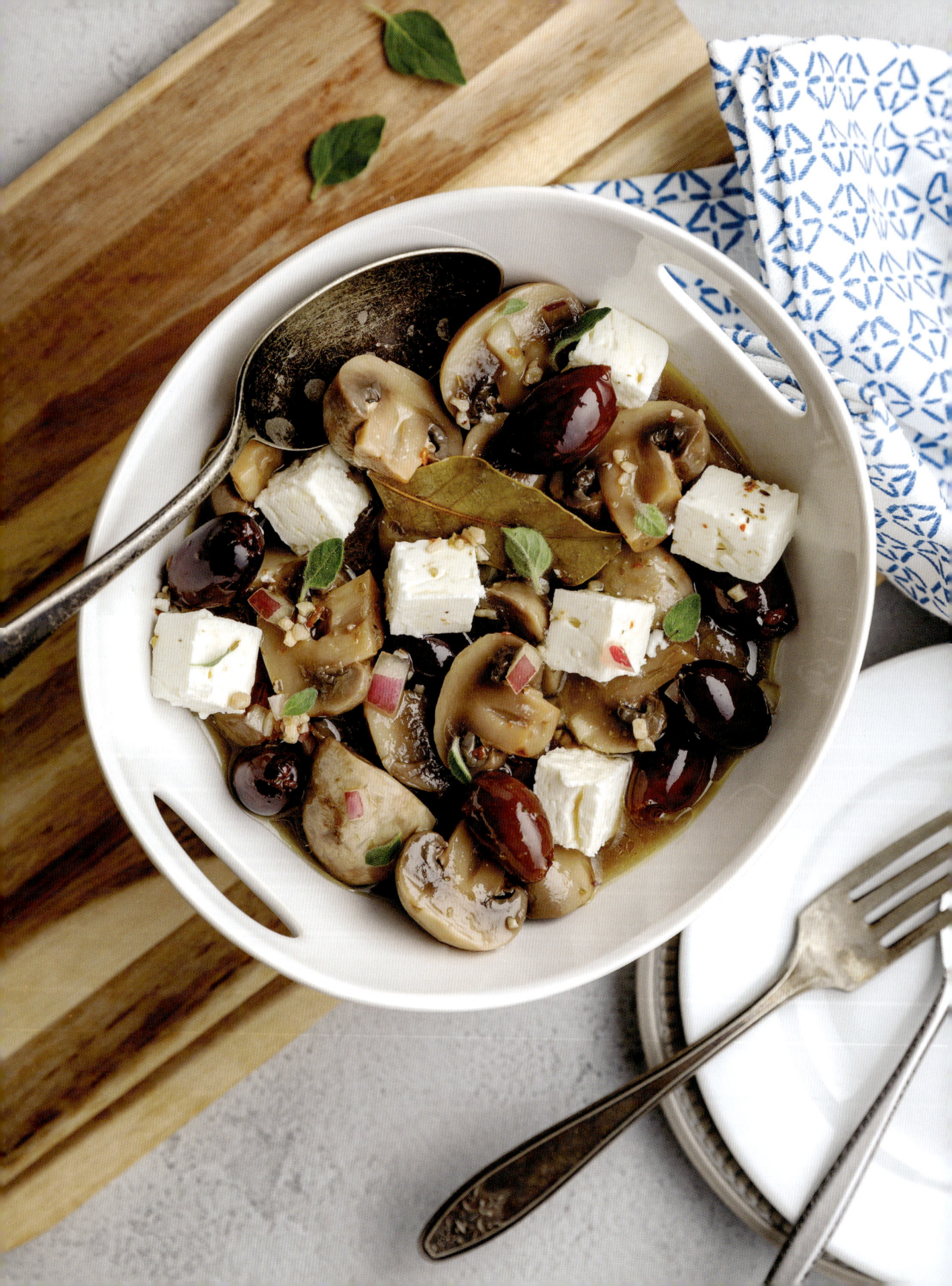

Prep Time: 10 min | High Pressure: 1 min | Quick Release | Serves: 6

# Greek Marinated Mushrooms

Lightly cooking these mushrooms under pressure infuses them with a Greek-style marinade in only a minute. It would take days to get this much flavor by marinating alone.

## Ingredients

16 ounces button mushrooms, halved

¼ cup white vinegar

¼ cup water

1 tablespoon minced garlic

2 teaspoons sugar substitute

1 bay leaf

½ teaspoon dried oregano

¼ teaspoon crushed red pepper flakes

½ cup kalamata olives, drained

2 tablespoons minced red onion

2 tablespoons extra-virgin olive oil

4 ounces cubed or crumbled feta cheese

Chopped fresh oregano, for garnish

Salt and pepper

1. Add mushrooms, vinegar, water, garlic, sugar substitute, bay leaf, dried oregano, and red pepper flakes to the Instant Pot and stir to combine.

2. Lock lid in place and seal pressure release vent. Set cooker to HIGH pressure for 1 minute.

3. Carefully open vent to quickly release the pressure.

4. Stir in kalamata olives, red onion, and olive oil. Cover and refrigerate at least 2 hours to continue marinating.

5. Stir in feta cheese and top with chopped fresh oregano before seasoning with salt and pepper to taste.

*Starters*

### Instant Tips

We add the feta cheese after chilling to ensure that it doesn't melt into the marinating liquid while the mushrooms are still warm.

Calories: 125 | Fat: 11g | Protein: 5.5g | Total Carbs: 4g - Fiber: 1.5g = Net Carbs: 2.5g

Instant Low Carb • 51

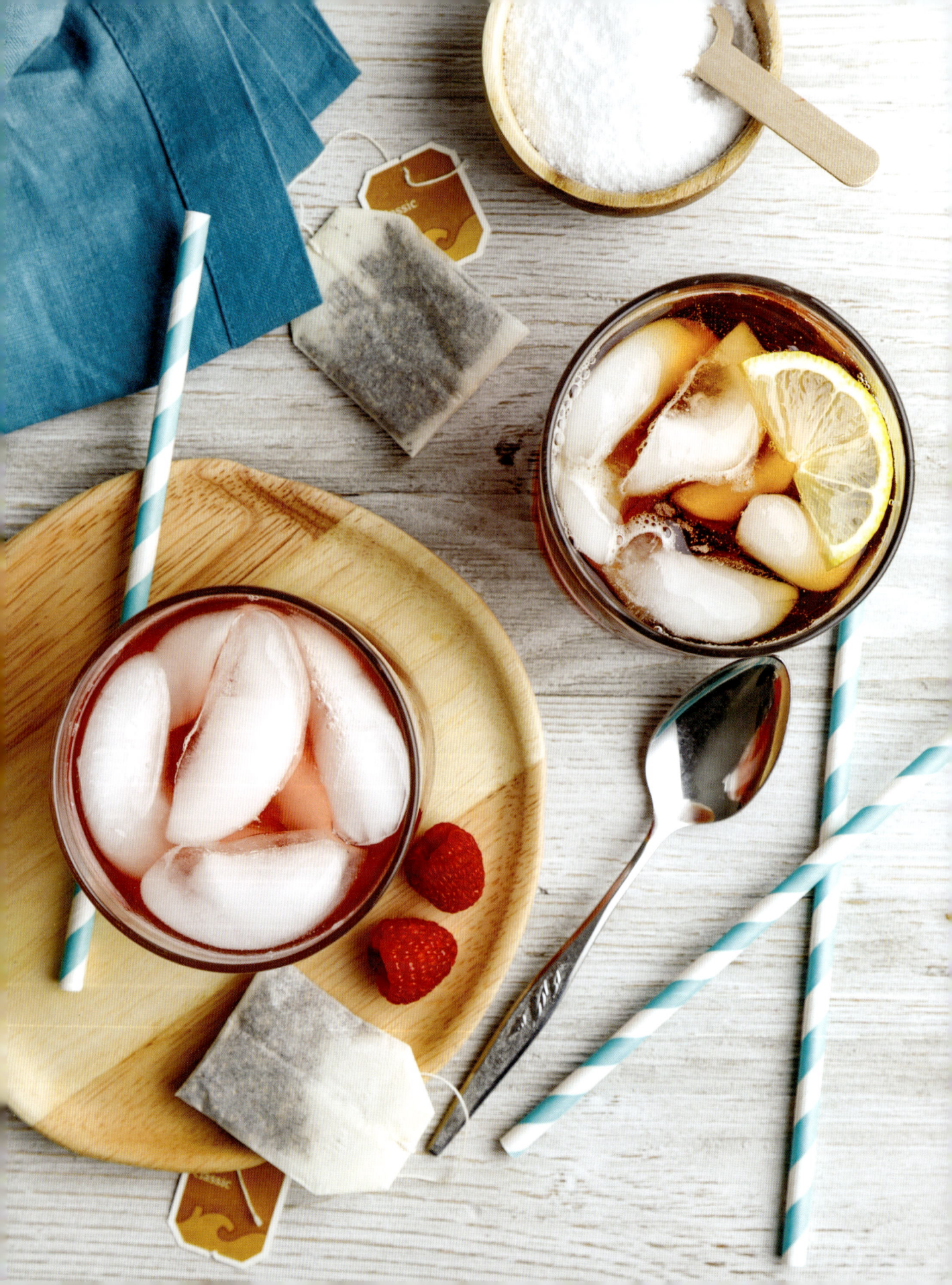

Prep Time: 5 min | High Pressure: 3 min | Natural Release: 20 min | Serves: 6

# Really Good Iced Tea

Pressure cooking tea isn't about saving time; it's about flavor and convenience. Boiling hot water can make tea bitter, but water does not come to a boil when heated under pressure, making for smooth tea that is robust and perfect for pouring over ice. You can even add fresh berries to infuse their flavor for homemade raspberry or blackberry iced tea. The juice from the berries does add their natural acidity, so be sure to sweeten those batches to taste. Nutrition provided is for 1 cup of raspberry-infused tea, as regular tea is basically free of calories and carbs.

## Ingredients

6 cups water

4 tea bags

½ cup fresh berries, optional

Sugar substitute to taste

## Special Equipment

Steam basket (optional)

1. For the easiest preparation (not required), insert a steam basket into the Instant Pot before pouring in water.

2. Remove any paper tags on the tea bags and submerge in the water.

3. For berry-infused tea, add berries.

4. Lock lid in place and seal pressure release vent. Set cooker to HIGH pressure for 3 minutes.

5. Let pressure release naturally for 20 minutes before opening vent to release any remaining pressure.

6. Grab the handle of the steam basket and remove from the tea, taking the tea bags and most of the fruit pulp with it. Discard tea bags and fruit pulp.

7. Let cool before pouring into a pitcher and storing refrigerated. For berry-infused tea, you can run it through a mesh strainer as you pour it into the pitcher to remove even more of the pulp.

8. Serve over a full glass of ice, sweetened with sugar substitute to taste.

**Instant Tips**

This works with any variety of tea, even hot tea when entertaining a crowd.

Calories: 5 | Fat: 0g | Protein: 0g | Total Carbs: 1g - Fiber: 0.5g = Net Carbs: 0.5g

Prep Time: 15 min | High Pressure: 4 min | Quick Release | Serves: 6

# Broccoli Cheese Dip

This creamy, cheesy spread with loads of broccoli is perfect for a platter or even just to dip into as a midday snack. Be warned, though—it can be hard to stop dipping once you've started! Celery sticks make the best low-carb dippers, but sliced zucchini works as well.

## Ingredients

1 cup chicken stock

2 cloves garlic

12 ounces broccoli florets (can use frozen)

8 ounces cream cheese, softened

1 cup shredded sharp Cheddar cheese

2 tablespoons minced yellow onion

1 tablespoon Dijon mustard

$1/2$ teaspoon Worcestershire sauce

Salt and pepper

## Special Equipment

Steam basket

1. Pour chicken stock into the Instant Pot and add garlic.
2. Insert steam basket over stock and add broccoli to the basket.
3. Lock lid in place and seal pressure release vent. Set cooker to HIGH pressure for 4 minutes.
4. Carefully open vent to quickly release the pressure.
5. Remove steam basket, reserve garlic from cooking liquid, and drain all cooking liquid.
6. Transfer the steamed broccoli and cooked garlic to the inner pot of the cooker and add all remaining ingredients.
7. Using a potato masher, mash the broccoli, cream cheese and other ingredients together to create a thick dip with most of the broccoli entirely mashed. Be sure to entirely mash the garlic cloves!
8. To heat the dip, set the cooker to SAUTÉ for just 1 minute before cancelling. Use a silicone spatula to constantly stir and ensure that none of the dip burns to the cooker. Repeat this process until heated through.
9. Season with salt and pepper to taste before serving with celery sticks or other low-carb dippers.

### Instant Tips

You can also mash the dip in a microwave-safe bowl, then microwave in 30-second intervals to heat it through without any risk of burning.

Calories: 190 | Fat: 14g | Protein: 9g | Total Carbs: 5g - Fiber: 1g = Net Carbs: 4g

Prep Time: 15 min | High Pressure: 0 min | Quick Release | Serves: 6

# Marinated Green Bean Antipasto

This cold Italian salad consists of snappy green beans that are marinated with salami and strips of provolone cheese, lightly tossed in olive oil and fresh basil. It makes for a great appetizer or even a light lunch.

## Ingredients

1 pound green beans, ends trimmed

¼ cup white wine vinegar

¼ cup water

1 tablespoon minced garlic

1 teaspoon sugar substitute

1 teaspoon Italian seasoning

4 ounces sliced salami, cut into strips

4 ounces sliced provolone cheese, cut into strips

¼ cup chopped fresh basil

2 tablespoons extra-virgin olive oil

Salt and pepper

1. Add green beans, vinegar, water, garlic, sugar substitute, and Italian seasoning to the Instant Pot and stir to combine.
2. Lock lid in place and seal pressure release vent. Set cooker to HIGH pressure for 0 minutes.
3. Carefully open vent to quickly release the pressure.
4. Let cool completely before stirring in all remaining ingredients.
5. Season with salt and pepper to taste before serving chilled.

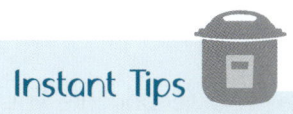

**Instant Tips**

This is also great with a combination of pepperoni, salami, and ham.

Calories: 190 | Fat: 14g | Protein: 10g | Total Carbs: 5.5g - Fiber: 2.5g = Net Carbs: 3g

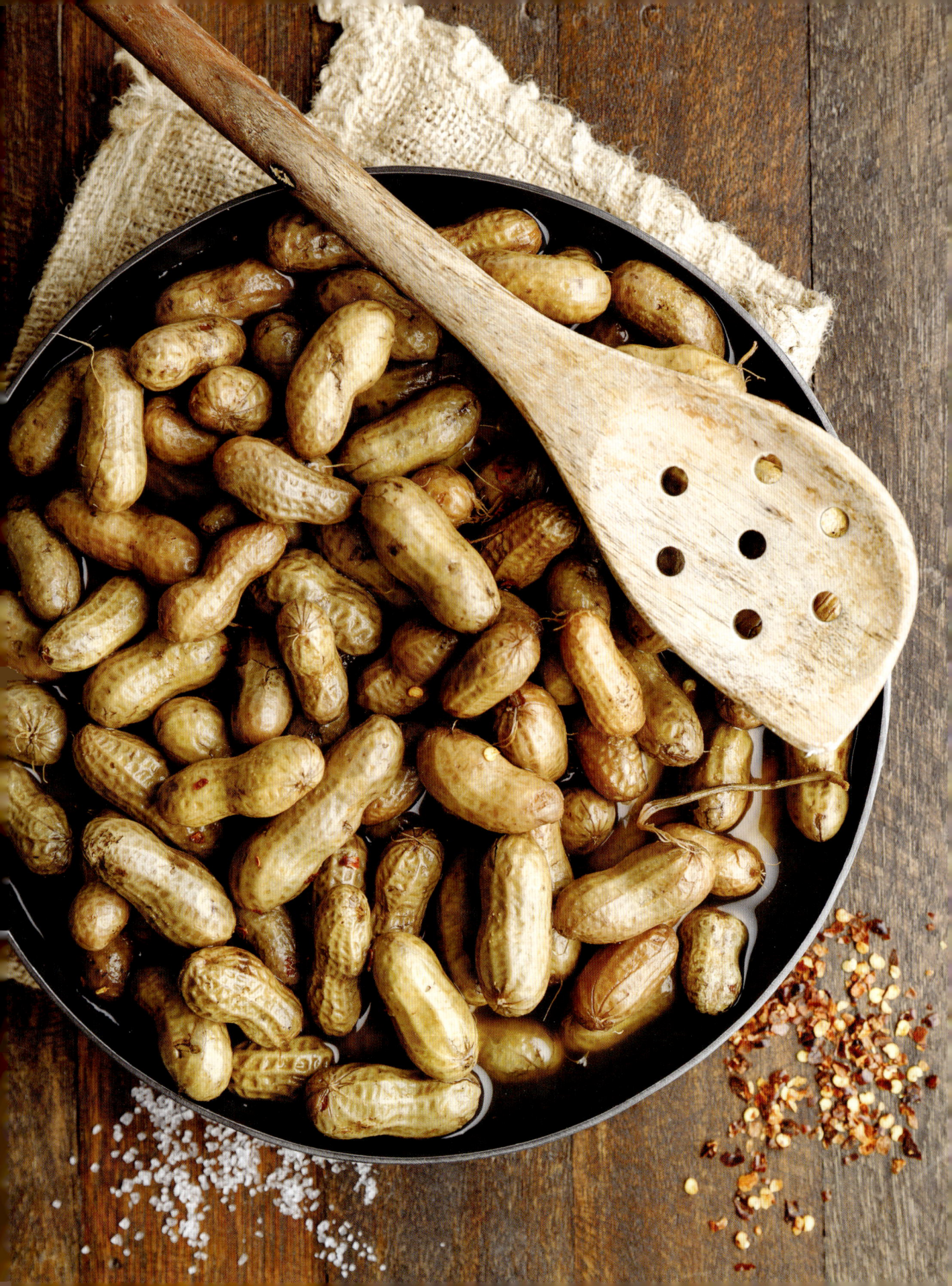

**Prep Time:** 5 min | **High Pressure:** 80 min | **Natural Release:** 15 min | **Serves:** 8

# Boiled Peanuts

Boiled peanuts are notorious for taking hours, if not the entire day, on the stove to cook up tender. Most recipes use the softer "green peanuts," which are sold refrigerated, to somewhat speed up the process, but the Instant Pot makes that unnecessary. In less time than traditionally boiling green peanuts takes, you can make this recipe from regular (unrefrigerated) raw peanuts. These unrefrigerated raw peanuts are usually larger, are available all year long, and typically cost 1/3 the price of fresh.

## Ingredients

1 pound raw peanuts (see tip)
1/2 cup kosher salt
2 teaspoons vegetable oil
2 teaspoons crushed red pepper flakes
1/2 teaspoon onion powder

## Special Equipment

Steam rack

1. Rinse peanuts and transfer to the Instant Pot.
2. Add enough water to the cooker to fully cover peanuts, then stir in salt, vegetable oil, pepper flakes, and onion powder.
3. Place the steam rack over the peanuts, then place a small heatproof ceramic plate over top the rack to weigh the peanuts down and keep them from floating.
4. Lock lid in place and seal pressure release vent. Set cooker to HIGH pressure for 80 minutes.
5. Let pressure release naturally for 15 minutes before opening vent to release any remaining pressure.
6. Serve warm or chilled. Store refrigerated in the cooking liquid.

### Instant Tips

The type of raw peanuts (not roasted) needed for the cook time in this recipe are sold unrefrigerated in large bags labeled "jumbo raw peanuts." Hampton Farms seems to be the main brand that sells them.

**Calories:** 260 | **Fat:** 23g | **Protein:** 12g | **Total Carbs:** 6.5g - **Fiber:** 4g = **Net Carbs:** 2.5g

Instant Low Carb • 57

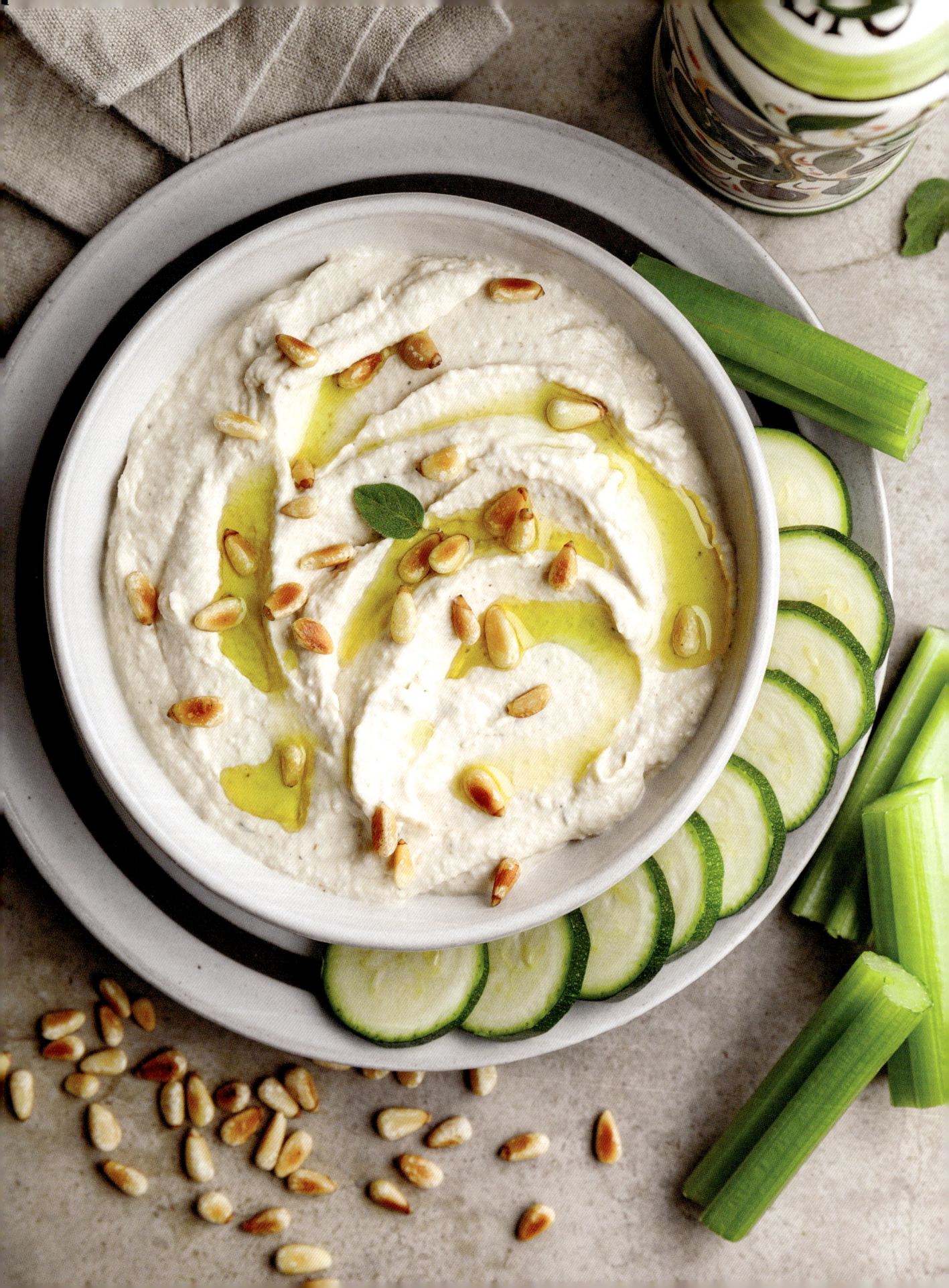

Prep Time: 10 min | High Pressure: 2 min | Quick Release | Serves: 6

# White "Bean" Dip with Pine Nuts

This taste of Tuscany is made with cauliflower florets rather than the cannellini beans typically used in ordinary white bean dip recipes. Much like legumes, cauliflower absorbs flavors, making it the perfect base for a smooth and creamy dip.

## Ingredients

1 cup vegetable stock

12 ounces cauliflower florets (about 3 cups)

4 ounces cream cheese

1/4 cup toasted pine nuts (see tip)

1 teaspoon lemon juice

3/4 teaspoon Italian seasoning

1/2 teaspoon sugar substitute

1/2 teaspoon salt

1/4 teaspoon pepper

1/4 teaspoon garlic powder

Extra-virgin olive oil, to top

## Special Equipment

Steam basket

1. Pour vegetable stock into the Instant Pot.
2. Insert steam basket over stock and add cauliflower to the basket.
3. Lock lid in place and seal pressure release vent. Set cooker to HIGH pressure for 2 minutes.
4. Carefully open vent to quickly release the pressure.
5. Transfer cauliflower to a food processor and add all remaining ingredients except olive oil. Discard cooking liquid from cooker.
6. Process dip until completely smooth. Cover and refrigerate.
7. Serve chilled with extra-virgin olive oil drizzled over the top. Serve with celery sticks or sliced zucchini for dipping.

### Instant Tips

You can now find toasted pine nuts for sale in some stores, but toasting your own is quite easy: Simply place in a sauté pan over medium heat and cook until golden brown and fragrant, about 5 minutes. Be sure to shake the pan from time to time as they cook for even toasting.

Calories: 100 | Fat: 8.5g | Protein: 3g | Total Carbs: 4.5g - Fiber: 1.5g = Net Carbs: 3g

Prep Time: 5 min | High Pressure: 20 min | Quick Release | Serves: 6

# Teriyaki Chicken Wings

These chicken wings are pressure-infused with a light teriyaki sauce (not glaze) that gives them a ton of flavor without drowning them in a ton of sticky, sugary sauce.

## Ingredients

- ½ cup teriyaki sauce (see tip)
- 2 tablespoons sugar substitute
- 2 teaspoons minced garlic
- 2 teaspoons grated ginger
- 1 tablespoon sesame oil
- 2 pounds frozen chicken wings

1. Add all ingredients except chicken wings to the Instant Pot and whisk to combine.
2. Add chicken wings to the sauce and toss to lightly coat wings.
3. Lock lid in place and seal pressure release vent. Set cooker to HIGH pressure for 20 minutes.
4. Carefully open vent to quickly release the pressure.
5. Toss cooked wings in the cooking liquid before transferring to a sheet pan. Drizzle a small amount of cooking liquid over top each wing.
6. Place under broiler for 5 minutes, just until chicken skin begins to crisp. Flip wings and drizzle with additional cooking liquid. Broil this side of the wings for 5 minutes or until crisp.

### Instant Tips

Look for thin teriyaki sauce (the same consistency as soy sauce) with only 2g of carbs or less per serving. In a pinch, you can simply use reduced-sodium soy sauce.

Calories: 335 | Fat: 25g | Protein: 24g | Total Carbs: 3.5g - Fiber: 0g = Net Carbs: 3.5g

**Prep Time: 1 min** | **High Pressure: 5 min** | **Natural Release: 5 min** | **Makes: 6–12**

# Instant Hard-Boiled Eggs

As a low-carb staple ingredient, there is always a reason to keep plenty of eggs stocked in the fridge, as well as a good supply of hard-boiled eggs to snack on between meals. Hard-boiling under pressure makes for eggs that are easier to peel than when prepared on the stovetop, especially if you go straight from the Instant Pot to a bath of ice water.

## Ingredients

6–12 large eggs

## Special Equipment

Steam rack

1. Pour 1 cup of water into the Instant Pot and insert steam rack.
2. Carefully arrange eggs atop the steam rack, stacking them if needed.
3. Lock lid in place and seal pressure release vent. Set cooker to HIGH pressure for 5 minutes. Note: For creamier yolks, set to HIGH pressure for only 4 minutes.
4. Let pressure release naturally for 5 minutes before opening vent to release any remaining pressure.
5. Fill a large bowl with water and ice to create an ice bath.
6. Carefully transfer the cooked eggs (they are hot!) to the ice bath and let cool at least 5 minutes.
7. Eggs can be peeled immediately or chilled for peeling later.

### Instant Tips

They also sell egg racks that you can place inside your cooker to hold each egg in place. Honestly, we've never seen a reason to use anything other than a regular steam rack or even a steam basket. They work just fine!

**Calories: 70** | **Fat: 5g** | **Protein: 6g** | **Total Carbs: 0g** - **Fiber: 0g** = **Net Carbs: 0g**

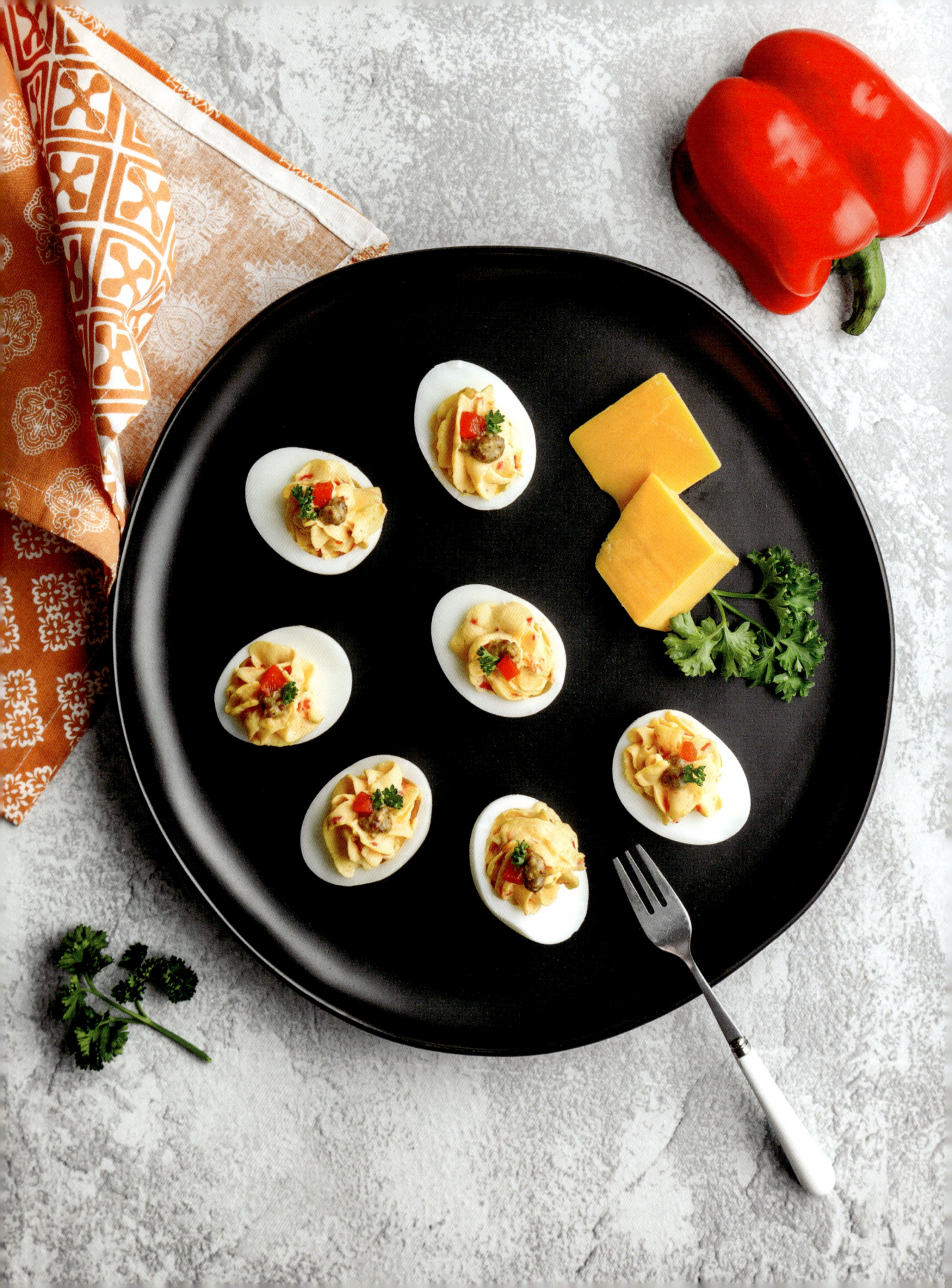

Prep Time: 20 min | Makes: 20 | Serves: 10

# Pimento-Cheese Deviled Eggs

Deviled eggs can be found on most party spreads down in the South, usually right beside a tub of pimento cheese dip, so it isn't too far a stretch to think that these two vastly different appetizers would go so well together.

## Ingredients

10 hard-boiled eggs (page: 61)
1/2 cup extra-sharp Cheddar cheese
3 tablespoons mayonnaise
1/2 teaspoon hot sauce
1/4 teaspoon paprika
1/4 teaspoon onion powder
1/4 teaspoon salt
1/4 cup diced pimentos, drained
2 tablespoons stone-ground mustard

### Special Equipment
Pastry bag (for best presentation)

1. Prepare and chill hard-boiled eggs before beginning.
2. Peel eggs and slice in half. Use a spoon to scoop the yolks into a food processor.
3. Add Cheddar cheese, mayonnaise, hot sauce, paprika, onion powder, and salt to the food processor and process until smooth.
4. Add diced pimentos to the food processor and pulse just until all is combined but with small bits of pimento intact throughout.
5. Transfer the pimento-cheese filling to a pastry bag or large food storage bag with the corner snipped off.
6. Pipe the filling evenly into the halves of each egg white.
7. Top each deviled egg with a very small dollop of stone-ground mustard before serving.

**Instant Tips**

For the best flavor, we always lightly salt the top of all egg whites before piping in the filling. This way the whites are as seasoned as the filling.

Calories: 125 | Fat: 10g | Protein: 7.5g | Total Carbs: 0.5g - Fiber: 0g = Net Carbs: 0.5g

*Chapter 3*

# Soups

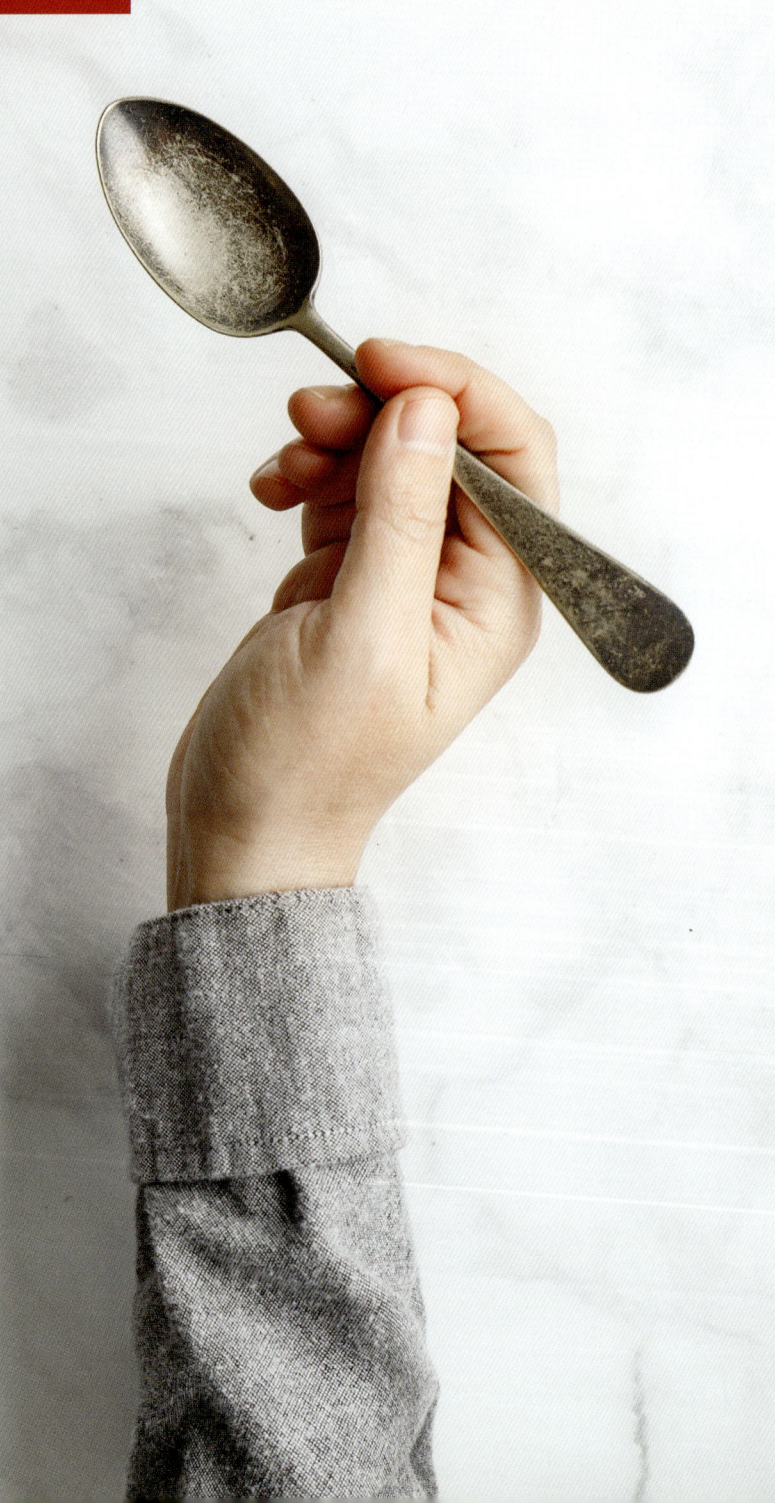

## recipes in this chapter...

**Chicken Noodle Soup, 67**

**Chicken Stock, 68**

**Chuck Roast Chili, 69**

**Cream of Mushroom Soup, 71**

**Creamy Cauliflower and Ham Soup, 72**

**Chicken Fajita Soup, 73**

**Chipotle Chili, 75**

**Polish Sausage and Cabbage Soup, 77**

**Italian Beef Stew, 78**

**Asparagus and Smoked Gouda Soup, 79**

**Tuscan Sausage Soup, 81**

**Chicken and Rice Soup, 82**

**Beef Burgundy Soup, 83**

**Creamy Tomato Soup, 85**

Secret Message #3: Christian has tons of silverware for photography but always reaches for the same few that are heavily tarnished in a beautiful way, though he wouldn't eat with them.

Instant Low Carb • 65

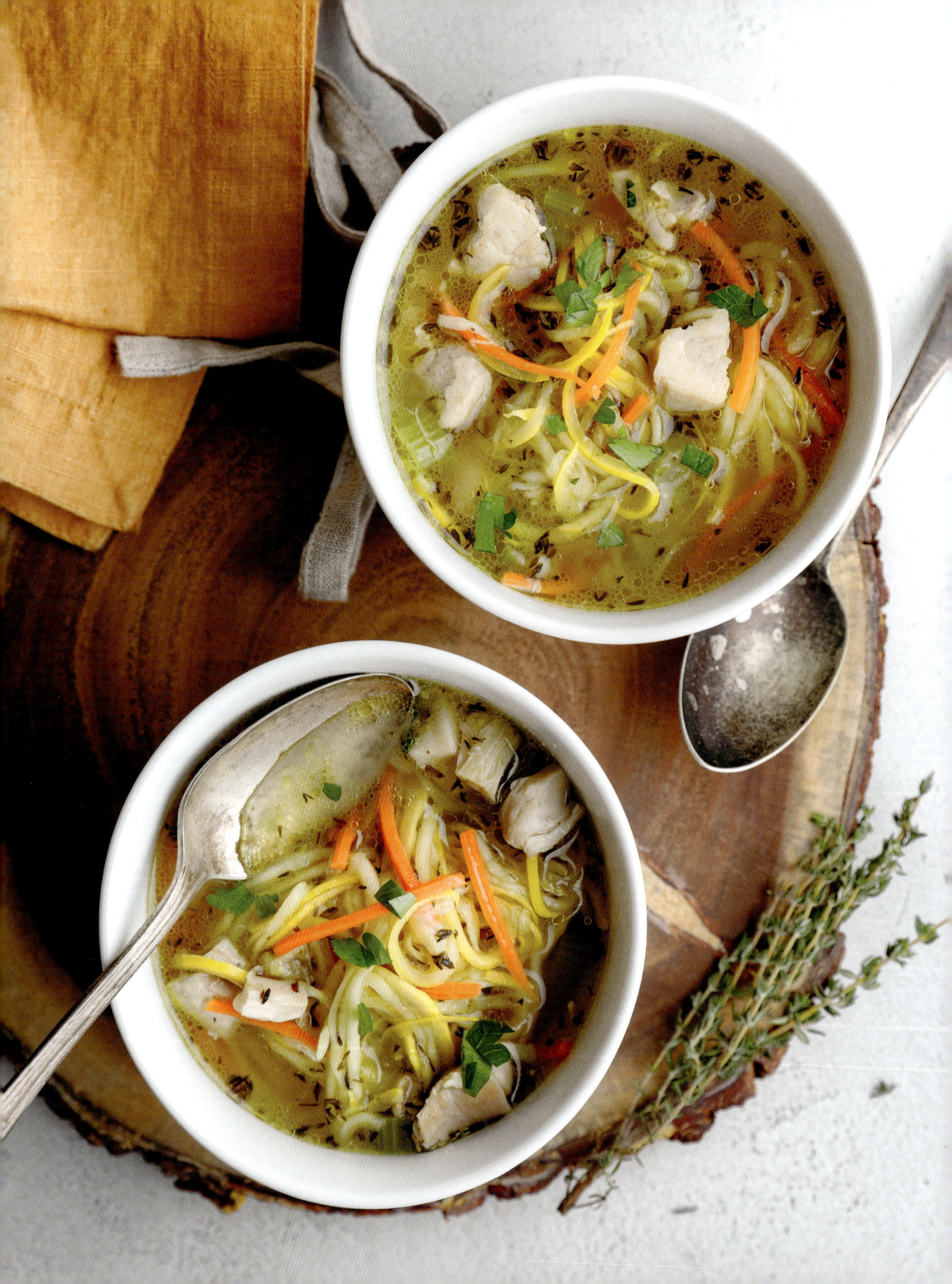

**Prep Time:** 15 min | **High Pressure:** 8 min | **Natural Release:** 5 min | **Serves:** 4

# Chicken Noodle Soup

Pressure cooking makes for extra-tender chicken in this classic soup, made low-carb thanks to spiralized yellow squash in place of traditional noodles.

## Ingredients

- 2 tablespoons olive oil
- 1 pound boneless, skinless chicken thighs, chopped
- Salt and pepper
- 1 cup chopped celery
- ½ cup diced yellow onion
- 2 teaspoons minced garlic
- 5 cups chicken stock
- 2 bay leaves
- ½ teaspoon dried thyme
- 4 cups spiralized yellow squash
- ¾ cup shredded carrots

1. Heat olive oil in the Instant Pot on the SAUTÉ setting.
2. Generously season chicken thighs with salt and pepper and add to the cooker, sautéing until they begin to lightly brown.
3. Add the celery, onion, and garlic and sauté 1 additional minute before stirring in chicken stock, bay leaves, and thyme.
4. Lock lid in place and seal pressure release vent. Set cooker to HIGH pressure for 8 minutes.
5. Let pressure release naturally for 5 minutes before opening vent to release any remaining pressure.
6. Stir in spiralized squash and shredded carrots and let rest for 1 minute to cook in the hot broth. Generously season soup with salt and pepper to taste before serving.

### Instant Tips

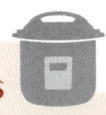

For even less carbs, simply omit the carrots or replace with matchstick-cut radishes. This will reduce carbs by about 2g.

**Calories:** 265 | **Fat:** 15g | **Protein:** 24.5g | **Total Carbs:** 9g - **Fiber:** 2.5g = **Net Carbs:** 6.5g

Instant Low Carb

**Prep Time: 10 min | High Pressure: 35 min | Natural Release: 20 min | Serves: 8**

# Chicken Stock

This method for making homemade chicken stock will leave you with a flavorful staple that can be used in any dish that calls for it (which is certainly a lot in this book). It makes for an especially soulful Chicken Noodle Soup, page: 67.

## Ingredients

Bones/carcass of 1 cooked chicken

2 cups vegetable scraps (celery and onions of any variety)

2 cloves garlic

1/2 teaspoon salt

1. Place chicken bones in the Instant Pot. It is great if there is still a little bit of meat left on the bones, but not necessary.
2. Add vegetable scraps, garlic, and salt.
3. Fill pot with water up to the max-fill line.
4. Lock lid in place and seal pressure release vent. Set cooker to HIGH pressure for 35 minutes.
5. Let pressure release naturally for 20 minutes before opening vent to release any remaining pressure.
6. Let cool before discarding all bones and vegetables.
7. Run the stock through a fine mesh strainer to remove any bits of meat or vegetables.
8. Store refrigerated for up to a week and frozen for up to 3 months.

### Instant Tips

Many people put fresh herbs in their chicken stock for more flavor, but we choose to leave that to the eventual dish the stock will be used to make.

**Calories: 70 | Fat: 3g | Protein: 7g | Total Carbs: 2g - Fiber: 0g = Net Carbs: 2g**

Prep Time: 20 min | High Pressure: 20 min | Natural Release: 15 min | Serves: 8

# Chuck Roast Chili

This chili is made from the same cut of beef you'd use to make pot roast, for a real hearty bowl with more texture than your typical ground beef chili.

## Ingredients

2 tablespoons olive oil

2 ½ pounds chuck roast, cut into ¾-inch cubes

1 small yellow onion, chopped

1 yellow bell pepper, chopped

1 jalapeño pepper, seeded and diced

3 tablespoons chili powder

1 tablespoon ground cumin

1 tablespoon minced garlic

1 teaspoon coriander

1 (14.5-ounce) can petite diced tomatoes, with liquid

1 cup beef stock

2 teaspoons sugar substitute

1 teaspoon salt

¾ teaspoon pepper

1 (8-ounce) can tomato sauce

¼ cup chopped fresh cilantro

1. Heat olive oil in the Instant Pot on the SAUTÉ setting.
2. Add chuck roast and sauté until it lightly browns.
3. Stir in onion, bell pepper, jalapeño, chili powder, cumin, minced garlic, and coriander and sauté 1 additional minute.
4. Stir in diced tomatoes, beef stock, sugar substitute, salt, and pepper.
5. Lock lid in place and seal pressure release vent. Set cooker to HIGH pressure for 20 minutes.
6. Let pressure release naturally for 15 minutes before opening vent to release any remaining pressure.
7. Set cooker to SAUTÉ and stir in tomato sauce and cilantro. Bring up to a simmer before serving.

### Instant Tips

For even more heat and a bit of crunch, we like to serve this topped with additional chopped jalapeño. For less heat, serve topped with fresh bell pepper.

Calories: 410 | Fat: 29g | Protein: 28.5g | Total Carbs: 7g - Fiber: 1.5g = Net Carbs: 5.5g

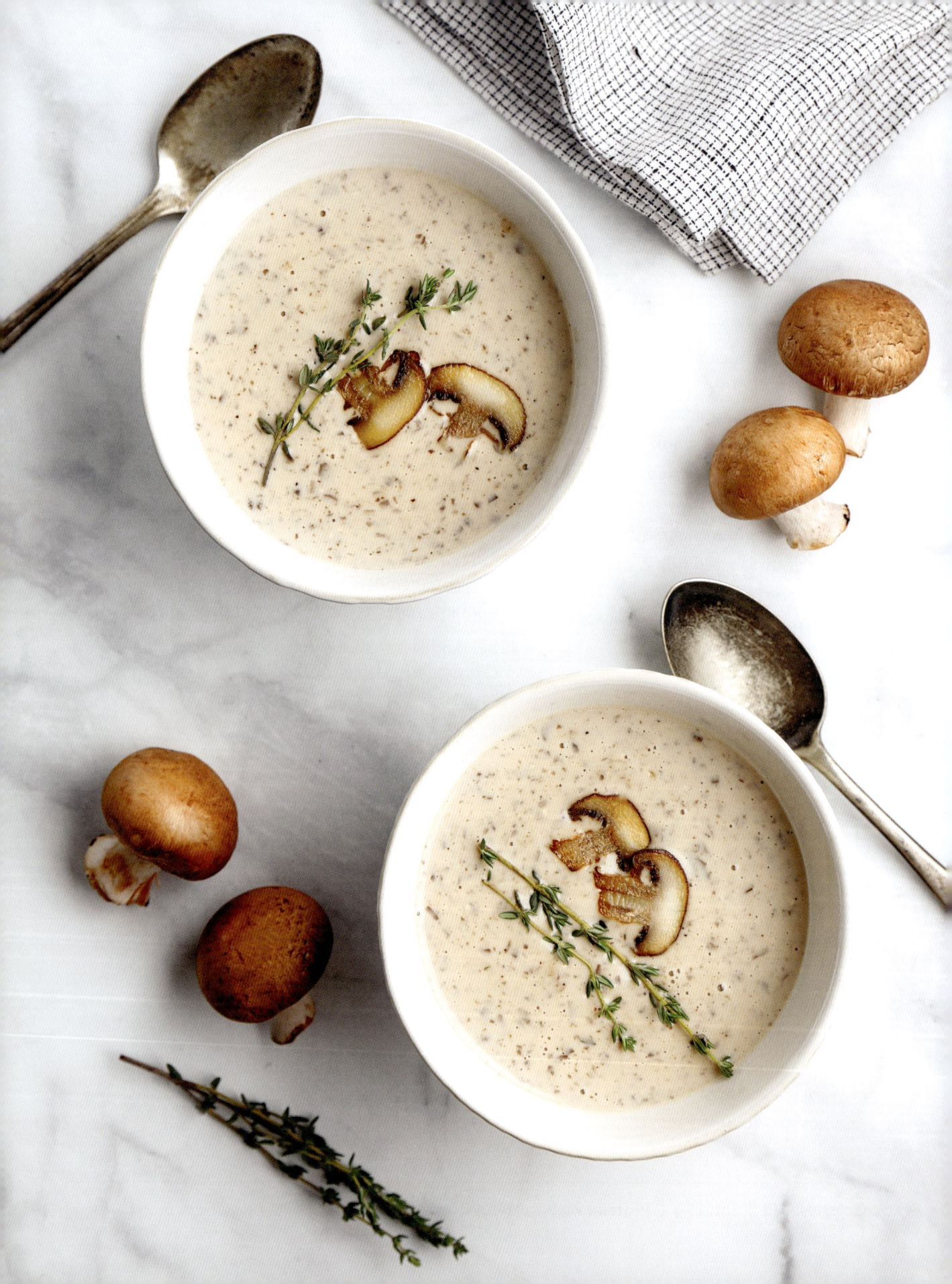

Prep Time: 15 min | High Pressure: 2 min | Quick Release | Serves: 6

# Cream of Mushroom Soup

The mushrooms in this classic soup practically melt right into the broth, making for a punch of flavor that would take a very, very long time to achieve on the stovetop.

## Ingredients

- 1 tablespoon vegetable oil
- 2 tablespoons butter
- 12 ounces baby bella mushrooms, minced (see tip)
- ½ cup diced yellow onion
- 2 teaspoons minced garlic
- 2 ½ cups beef stock
- 3 tablespoons sherry cooking wine
- 2 sprigs fresh thyme
- 1 bay leaf
- ¾ teaspoon celery salt
- ¾ teaspoon pepper
- 1 cup heavy cream
- 4 ounces cream cheese

1. Heat vegetable oil and butter in the Instant Pot on the SAUTÉ setting.
2. Add the mushrooms, onion, and garlic and sauté for 4 minutes or until onion begins to turn translucent.
3. Stir in beef stock, sherry, thyme, bay leaf, celery salt, and pepper.
4. Lock lid in place and seal pressure release vent. Set cooker to HIGH pressure for 2 minutes.
5. Carefully open vent to quickly release the pressure.
6. Set cooker to SAUTÉ and add heavy cream, bringing it up to a simmer. Stirring constantly, let simmer 5 minutes to slightly thicken.
7. Turn off the cooker and stir in cream cheese before serving.

**Instant Tips**

You can quickly mince the mushrooms by adding to a food processor and pulsing just a few times until they are finely chopped.

Calories: 285 | Fat: 29g | Protein: 4g | Total Carbs: 5g - Fiber: 1g = Net Carbs: 4g

Prep Time: 10 min | High Pressure: 3 min | Quick Release | Serves: 6

# Creamy Cauliflower and Ham Soup

This take on a loaded potato soup has everything you'd expect—except the potato! By using ham, you can skip the browning of (the more traditional) bacon.

## Ingredients

- 1 head cauliflower, chopped
- 2 cups chicken stock
- 1/2 cup diced yellow onion
- 1/2 teaspoon dried thyme
- 1/2 teaspoon salt
- 1/2 teaspoon pepper
- 8 ounces diced ham
- 1/2 cup heavy cream
- 1/2 cup sour cream
- 1/2 cup shredded sharp Cheddar cheese
- 2 scallions, sliced

1. Place cauliflower, chicken stock, onion, thyme, salt, and pepper in the Instant Pot and toss to combine.
2. Lock lid in place and seal pressure release vent. Set cooker to HIGH pressure for 3 minutes.
3. Carefully open vent to quickly release the pressure.
4. Use an immersion blender to fully purée the cauliflower until smooth. This can also be done by carefully transferring to a food processor or blender.
5. Set cooker to SAUTÉ and add ham and heavy cream. Bring up to a simmer.
6. Turn off heat and stir in sour cream before serving topped with shredded Cheddar cheese and sliced scallions.

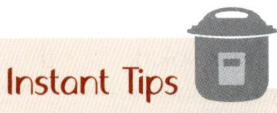

**Instant Tips**

This is also great with cooked and crumbled bacon in place of the ham.

Calories: 225 | Fat: 15.5g | Protein: 12g | Total Carbs: 9g - Fiber: 3g = Net Carbs: 6g

**Prep Time:** 15 min | **High Pressure:** 15 min | **Natural Release:** 5 min | **Serves:** 6

# Chicken Fajita Soup

This Southwestern soup has pulled chicken, two colors of bell pepper, red onion, and fresh cilantro—all your favorite fajita fixings! The broth is finished with cream cheese and Cheddar cheese to sub in for the creaminess of sour cream and shredded cheese in traditional fajitas.

## Ingredients

- 3 boneless, skinless chicken breasts
- 3 cups chicken stock
- 1 cup jarred salsa
- 1 tablespoon chili powder
- 2 teaspoons ground cumin
- ¾ teaspoon salt
- ¾ teaspoon pepper
- ½ red bell pepper, diced
- ½ green bell pepper, diced
- ½ cup diced red onion
- 8 ounces cream cheese, chopped
- 1 cup sharp Cheddar cheese
- ¼ cup chopped fresh cilantro

1. Place chicken, chicken stock, salsa, chili powder, cumin, salt, and pepper in the Instant Pot and stir to combine.
2. Lock lid in place and seal pressure release vent. Set cooker to HIGH pressure for 15 minutes.
3. Let pressure release naturally for 5 minutes before opening vent to release any remaining pressure.
4. Remove chicken from cooker and set aside.
5. Set cooker to SAUTÉ and stir in bell peppers and red onion, bringing them up to a simmer. Simmer for 5 minutes or until tender.
6. As the soup is simmering, use two forks to pull the chicken into bite-sized shreds.
7. Turn off cooker and stir in cream cheese and shredded chicken. Once the cream cheese has mostly melted into the soup, stir in Cheddar cheese and cilantro until all is combined. Serve immediately.

### Instant Tips

You can also make this by adding the peppers and onion before pressure cooking, but they will almost melt into the broth. It makes for good flavor, but we prefer the texture using the method above.

**Calories:** 290 | **Fat:** 18.5g | **Protein:** 20g | **Total Carbs:** 8g  -  **Fiber:** 2g  =  **Net Carbs:** 6g

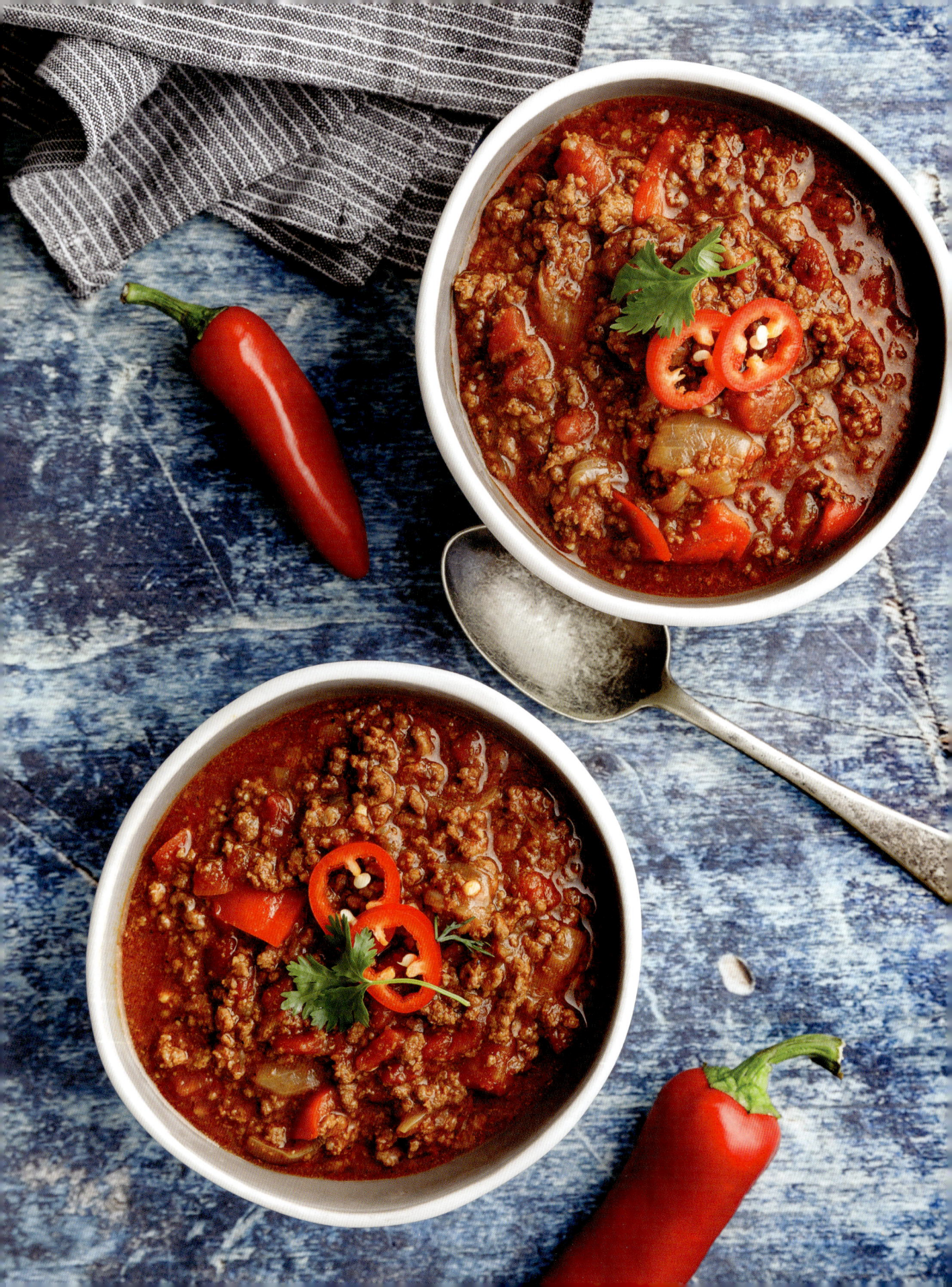

**Prep Time:** 15 min | **High Pressure:** 5 min | **Natural Release:** 15 min | **Serves:** 6

# Chipotle Chili

We've added a bit of smokiness as well as a Tex-Mex flare to this low-carb ground beef chili. It is perfect for when cooler weather rolls around and you need a big bowl of warmth with a good kick of spice. Did we mention that this is spicy?

## Ingredients

- 1 tablespoon olive oil
- 1 1/2 pounds ground beef
- 1 small yellow onion, chopped
- 1 red bell pepper, chopped
- 2 tablespoons chipotle chili powder
- 1 tablespoon smoked paprika
- 1 tablespoon ground cumin
- 1 tablespoon minced garlic
- 1 teaspoon dried oregano
- 1 (14.5-ounce) can petite diced tomatoes, with liquid
- 1 1/4 cups beef stock
- 2 tablespoons tomato paste
- 1 teaspoon salt
- 3/4 teaspoon pepper

1. Heat olive oil in the Instant Pot on the SAUTÉ setting.
2. Add ground beef and crumble it as it browns. Drain excess grease.
3. Stir in onion, bell pepper, chili powder, paprika, cumin, minced garlic, and oregano and sauté 1 additional minute.
4. Stir in all remaining ingredients.
5. Lock lid in place and seal pressure release vent. Set cooker to HIGH pressure for 5 minutes.
6. Let pressure release naturally for 15 minutes before opening vent to release any remaining pressure.
7. Let cool for 5 minutes to thicken slightly before serving.

**Instant Tips**

This recipe can be used to make traditional low-carb chili by substituting regular chili powder and regular paprika in place of the chipotle chili powder and smoked paprika.

**Calories:** 290 | **Fat:** 19.5g | **Protein:** 22g | **Total Carbs:** 6.5g - **Fiber:** 1.5g = **Net Carbs:** 5g

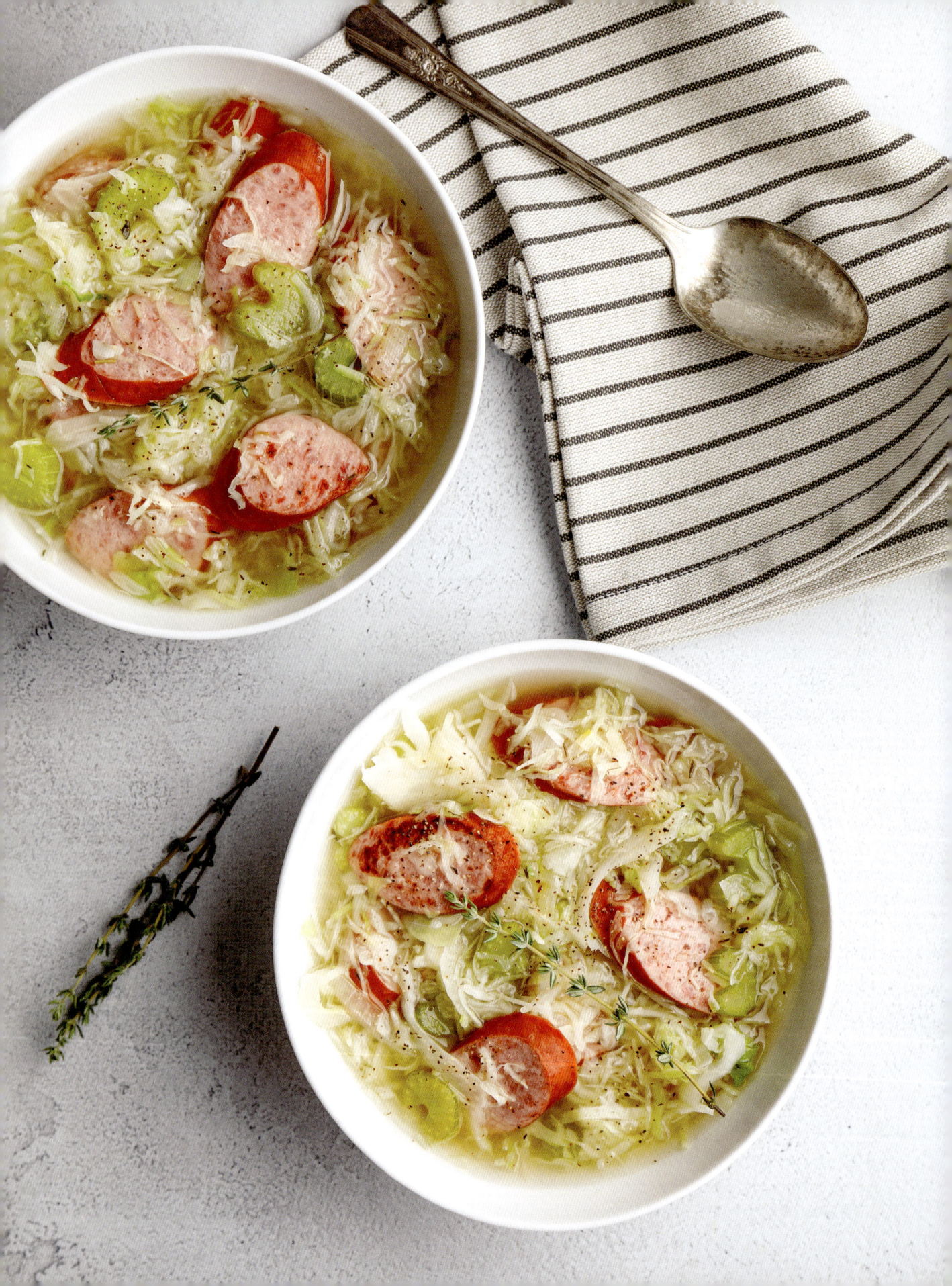

Prep Time: 15 min | High Pressure: 2 min | Quick Release | Serves: 6

# Polish Sausage and Cabbage Soup

The classic combination of sausage and cabbage makes for a simple dish that's a light and refreshing change from chicken or beef-based soups.

## Ingredients

1 tablespoon vegetable oil

1 tablespoon butter

12–14 ounces smoked Polish sausage, sliced or large chopped

1 small yellow onion, thinly sliced

3 stalks celery, chopped

4 cups shredded green cabbage

5 cups chicken stock

2 tablespoons white vinegar

2 teaspoons sugar substitute

½ teaspoon dried thyme

½ teaspoon onion powder

1 bay leaf

½ teaspoon salt

½ teaspoon pepper

1. Heat vegetable oil and butter in the Instant Pot on the SAUTÉ setting.
2. Add the sausage, onion, and celery and sauté 4 minutes or until onion begins to sweat.
3. Stir in all remaining ingredients.
4. Lock lid in place and seal pressure release vent. Set cooker to HIGH pressure for 2 minutes.
5. Carefully open vent to quickly release the pressure. Serve immediately.

**Instant Tips**

This is really good with a splash of hot sauce added at the table.

Calories: 230 | Fat: 17.5g | Protein: 13g | Total Carbs: 5g - Fiber: 1.5g = Net Carbs: 3.5g

**Prep Time:** 15 min | **High Pressure:** 25 min | **Natural Release:** 15 min | **Serves:** 6

# Italian Beef Stew

Chunks of beef are stewed in a hearty tomato-based broth with tender zucchini, making a bowl of this Italian-stew satisfying enough to make a complete meal.

## Ingredients

- 2 tablespoons olive oil
- 2 pounds beef stew meat
- 1 small red onion, chopped large
- 4 stalks celery, chopped large
- 1 tablespoon minced garlic
- 1 (14.5-ounce) can petite diced tomatoes, with liquid
- 2 cups beef stock
- 2 teaspoons Italian seasoning
- 1 teaspoon salt
- 1 teaspoon pepper
- ¼ teaspoon crushed red pepper flakes
- 2 zucchini, chopped

1. Heat olive oil in the Instant Pot on the SAUTÉ setting.
2. Add stew meat and sauté until it lightly browns.
3. Stir in onion, celery, and minced garlic and sauté 1 additional minute.
4. Stir in diced tomatoes, beef stock, Italian seasoning, salt, pepper, and crushed red pepper flakes.
5. Lock lid in place and seal pressure release vent. Set cooker to HIGH pressure for 25 minutes.
6. Let pressure release naturally for 15 minutes before opening vent to release any remaining pressure.
7. Set cooker to SAUTÉ and stir in zucchini. Let simmer 5 minutes or until zucchini is tender.

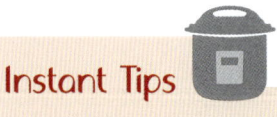

**Instant Tips**

For a slightly thicker stew, stir in 1 to 2 tablespoons of tomato paste when you add the zucchini.

**Calories:** 350 | **Fat:** 23g | **Protein:** 28g | **Total Carbs:** 6.5g - **Fiber:** 1.5g = **Net Carbs:** 5g

Prep Time: 10 min | High Pressure: 10 min | Quick Release | Serves: 4

# Asparagus and Smoked Gouda Soup

Cream of asparagus soup is all grown up in this recipe thanks to the addition of smoked gouda, which lends a mild and mature flavor that doesn't overpower the asparagus.

## Ingredients

1 pound asparagus, ends trimmed

2 cups chicken stock

1/2 cup diced yellow onion

2 teaspoons minced garlic

1 bay leaf

1/2 teaspoon salt

1/2 teaspoon pepper

1/2 cup heavy cream

1 cup shredded smoked gouda cheese

1. Place asparagus, chicken stock, onion, garlic, bay leaf, salt, and pepper in the Instant Pot and stir to combine.

2. Lock lid in place and seal pressure release vent. Set cooker to HIGH pressure for 10 minutes.

3. Carefully open vent to quickly release the pressure. Discard bay leaf.

4. Use an immersion blender to fully purée the asparagus until smooth. This can also be done by carefully transferring to a food processor or blender.

5. Set cooker to SAUTÉ and stir in heavy cream, bringing the soup up to a simmer.

6. Turn off heat and stir in smoked gouda cheese before serving.

### Instant Tips

For the best presentation, cut and reserve a few asparagus tips before pressure cooking. Cover and microwave for 1 minute or until tender before using to garnish the finished soup.

Calories: 230 | Fat: 19g | Protein: 9.5g | Total Carbs: 6.5g  -  Fiber: 2.5g  =  Net Carbs: 4g

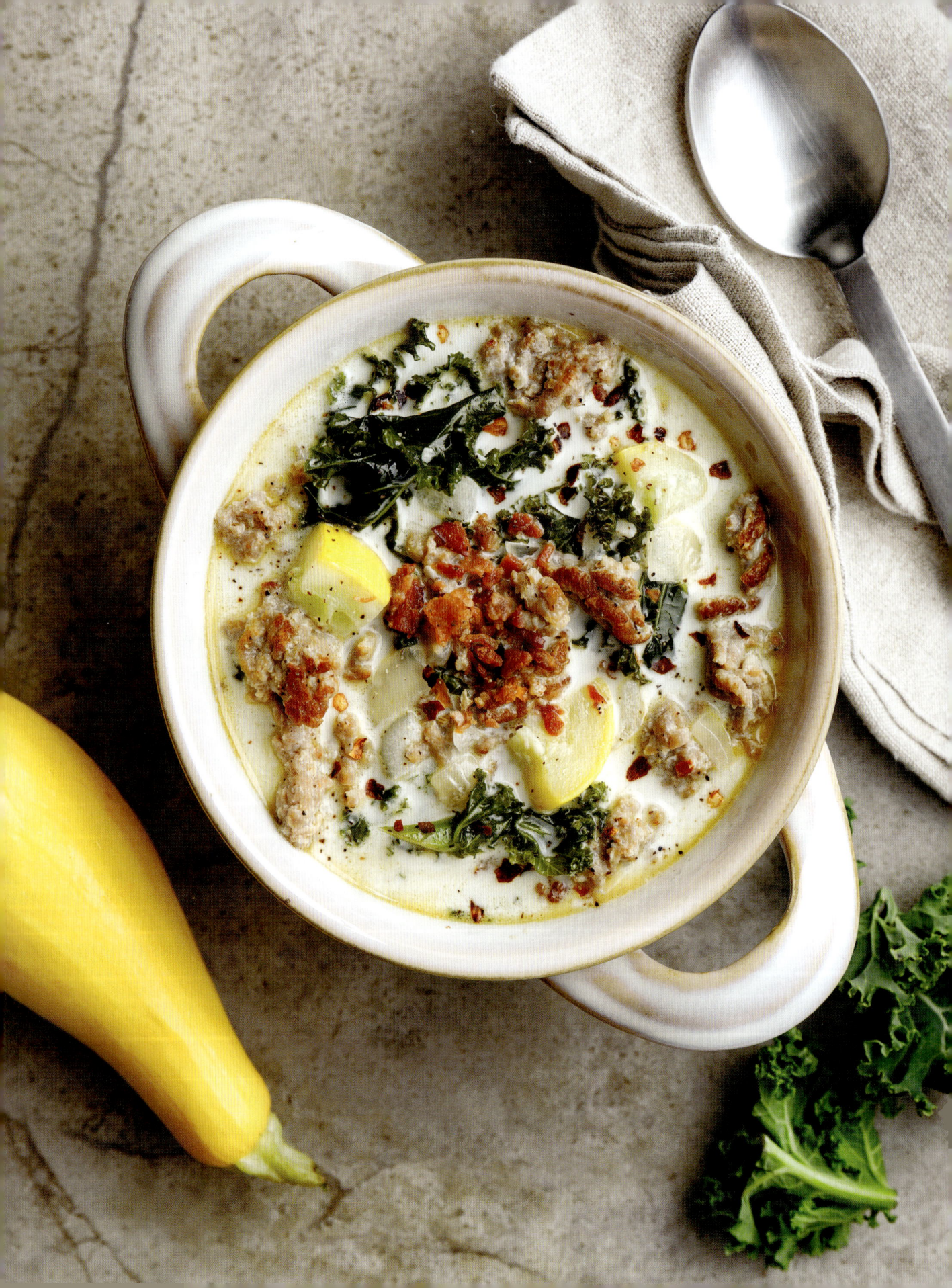

Prep Time: 10 min | High Pressure: 5 min | Quick Release | Serves: 6

# Tuscan Sausage Soup

The flavors of faux-Italy combine in this copy of a famous Italian chain-restaurant's "Toscana" soup. It might not have been our idea to combine bacon, Italian sausage, and kale in a light (and somewhat spicy!) broth with a touch of cream, but we will admit that it was a very good idea. Our only major change is that we use chopped yellow squash in place of potatoes.

## Ingredients

- 1 tablespoon olive oil
- 3 slices bacon, finely diced
- 1 pound ground Italian sausage
- ½ cup diced yellow onion
- 1 tablespoon minced garlic
- 4 cups vegetable stock
- 4 cups chopped kale
- 1 bay leaf
- ½ teaspoon crushed red pepper flakes
- ¼ teaspoon salt
- ¼ teaspoon pepper
- 2 yellow squash, chopped
- 1 cup heavy cream

1. Heat olive oil and bacon in the Instant Pot on the SAUTÉ setting, just until bacon begins to crisp.
2. Add the sausage and crumble it as it browns.
3. Add the onion and garlic and sauté 1 additional minute before draining excess grease.
4. Stir in vegetable stock, kale, bay leaf, red pepper flakes, salt, and pepper.
5. Lock lid in place and seal pressure release vent. Set cooker to HIGH pressure for 5 minutes.
6. Carefully open vent to quickly release the pressure.
7. Set cooker to SAUTÉ and add squash and heavy cream.
8. Let simmer 5 minutes, stirring occasionally, until squash has softened.

### Instant Tips

This is best when served topped with shredded Parmesan cheese.

Calories: 450 | Fat: 36g | Protein: 23g | Total Carbs: 7.5g - Fiber: 2.5g = Net Carbs: 5g

Prep Time: 15 min | High Pressure: 8 min | Natural Release: 5 min | Serves: 6

# Chicken and Rice Soup

There really isn't any reason to buy high-carb canned soup when the Instant Pot makes an amazingly flavorful soup in just minutes and with minimal effort. For the "rice," we used grated cauliflower that you add to the creamy broth after pressure cooking to ensure it retains its texture.

## Ingredients

- 1 tablespoon vegetable oil
- 1 tablespoon butter
- 1 pound boneless, skinless chicken thighs, chopped
- Salt and pepper
- 1 cup chopped celery
- 1/2 cup diced red onion
- 2 teaspoons minced garlic
- 4 cups chicken stock
- 3 sprigs fresh thyme
- 1/2 teaspoon poultry seasoning
- 1/2 cup heavy cream
- 2 cups grated cauliflower (cauliflower rice)
- 1/4 cup diced red bell pepper

1. Heat vegetable oil and butter in the Instant Pot on the SAUTÉ setting.
2. Generously season chicken thighs with salt and pepper and add to the cooker, sautéing until they begin to lightly brown.
3. Add the celery, onion, and garlic and sauté 1 additional minute before stirring in chicken stock, thyme, and poultry seasoning.
4. Lock lid in place and seal pressure release vent. Set cooker to HIGH pressure for 8 minutes.
5. Let pressure release naturally for 5 minutes before opening vent to release any remaining pressure.
6. Set cooker to SAUTÉ and stir in heavy cream, cauliflower rice, and bell pepper. Bring up to a simmer and cook 5 minutes or until cauliflower is crisp-tender.
7. Generously season soup with salt and pepper to taste before serving.

### Instant Tips

This can be made with shredded chicken breasts, using 1 pound of boneless, skinless chicken breasts and increasing the time under pressure to 15 minutes. Then, shred the chicken into the broth.

Calories: 230 | Fat: 17.5g | Protein: 15.5g | Total Carbs: 3.5g - Fiber: 0.5g = Net Carbs: 3g

Prep Time: 20 min | High Pressure: 25 min | Natural Release: 15 min | Serves: 6

# Beef Burgundy Soup

This hearty soup with tender chunks of beef, fresh vegetables, and herbs in a red wine broth tastes like it has been stewing all day, when in fact it takes less than half an hour under pressure.

## Ingredients

- 3 slices bacon, chopped
- 2 pounds beef stew meat
- 8 ounces button mushrooms, halved
- 1/2 cup chopped yellow onion
- 3 stalks celery, chopped large
- 1 tablespoon minced garlic
- 2 1/2 cups beef stock
- 1 cup dry red wine
- 2 tablespoons tomato paste
- 3 sprigs fresh thyme
- 1 bay leaf
- 1 teaspoon salt
- 1 teaspoon pepper
- 3/4 teaspoon onion powder
- 2 large yellow squash, sliced into ribbons

1. Heat bacon in the Instant Pot on the SAUTÉ setting until nearly crisp.
2. Add stew meat and sauté until it starts to lightly brown.
3. Stir in mushrooms, onion, celery, and minced garlic and sauté 1 additional minute.
4. Stir in all remaining ingredients except yellow squash.
5. Lock lid in place and seal pressure release vent. Set cooker to HIGH pressure for 25 minutes.
6. Let pressure release naturally for 15 minutes before opening vent to release any remaining pressure.
7. Set cooker to SAUTÉ and stir in yellow squash. Let simmer 3 minutes or until squash is crisp-tender.

**Instant Tips**
Add another splash of wine when you add the squash to wake up that vino flavor!

Calories: 370 | Fat: 21g | Protein: 30g | Total Carbs: 7g - Fiber: 2g = Net Carbs: 5g

Instant Low Carb • 83

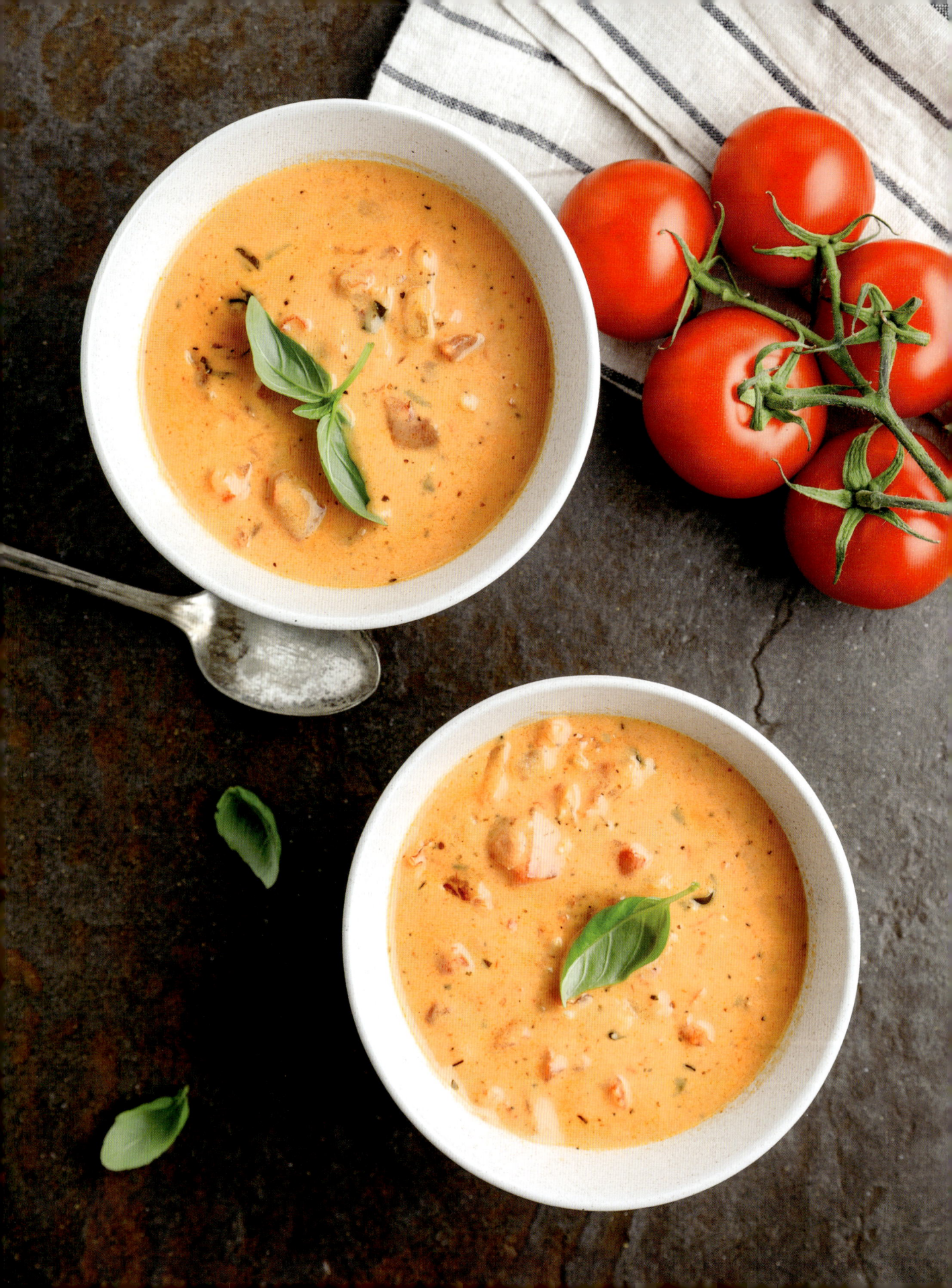

Prep Time: 10 min | High Pressure: 5 min | Natural Release: 5 min | Serves: 6

# Creamy Tomato Soup

Most versions of this classic soup contain a good amount of added sugar and a ton of natural sugars from various tomato products. We use less tomato to keep those natural sugars down but then pressure cook to ensure their flavor is throughout the broth.

## Ingredients

- 2 tablespoons butter
- 1/2 cup diced yellow onion
- 2 teaspoons minced garlic
- 1 (14.5-ounce) can petite diced tomatoes, with liquid
- 2 1/2 cups chicken stock
- 3 tablespoons tomato paste
- 1 teaspoon Italian seasoning
- 1 teaspoon sugar substitute
- 1/2 teaspoon salt
- 1/2 teaspoon pepper
- 3/4 cup heavy cream
- 1/4 cup chopped fresh basil

1. Heat butter in the Instant Pot on the SAUTÉ setting.
2. Add the onion and garlic and sauté for 4 minutes or until onions begin to turn translucent.
3. Stir in all remaining ingredients except heavy cream and basil.
4. Lock lid in place and seal pressure release vent. Set cooker to HIGH pressure for 5 minutes.
5. Let pressure release naturally for 5 minutes before opening vent to let out any remaining pressure.
6. Stir in heavy cream and basil before serving.

### Instant Tips

For even more flavor, let the soup simmer, stirring constantly, for 5 minutes after adding the heavy cream but before adding the basil.

Calories: 170 | Fat: 16g | Protein: 1.5g | Total Carbs: 7g - Fiber: 1g = Net Carbs: 6g

Instant Low Carb • 85

Chapter 4

# *Poultry*

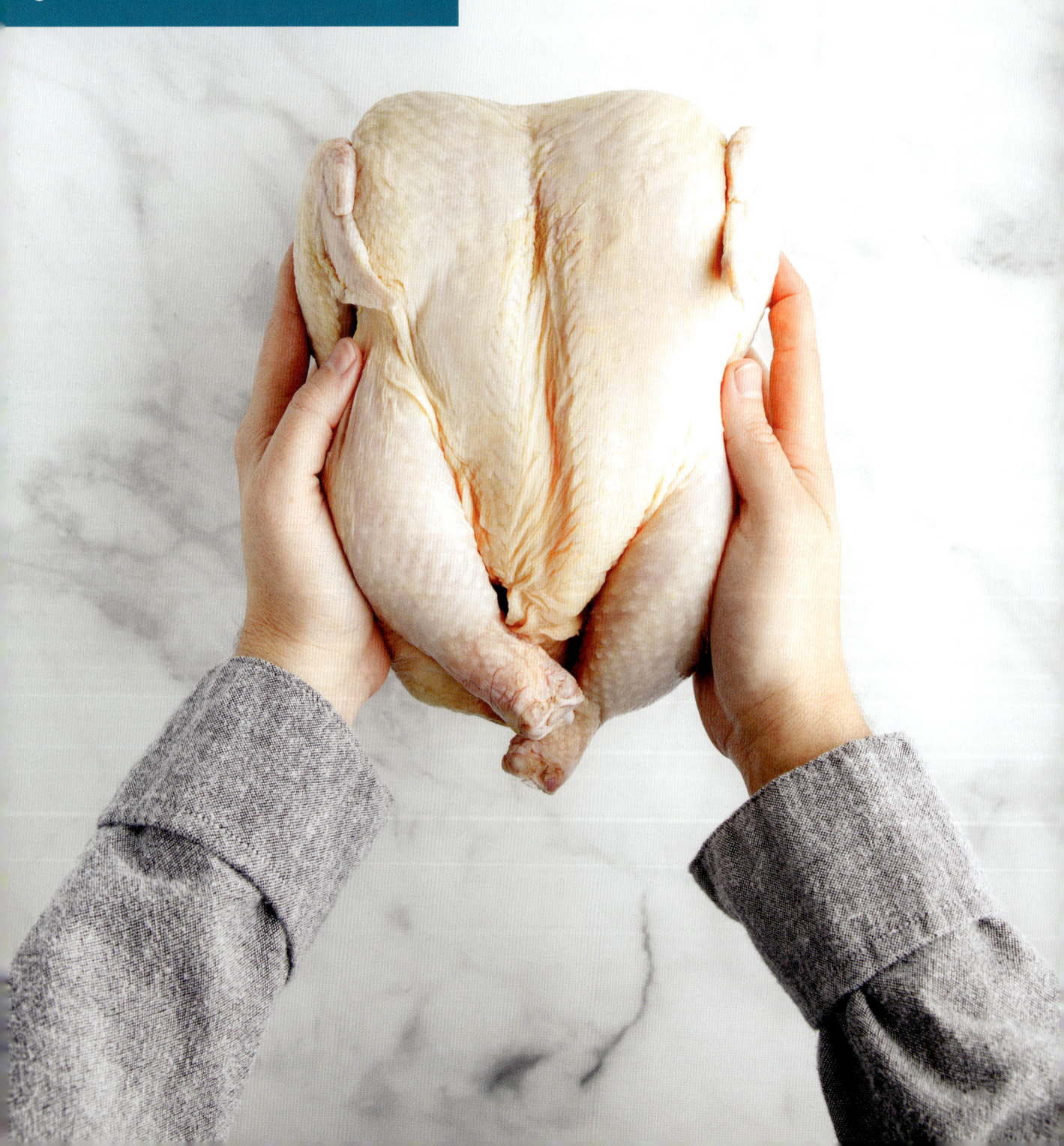

## recipes in this chapter...

**Chicken Parmesan, 89**

**Indian Butter Chicken, 91**

**Honey Mustard Chicken Drumsticks, 92**

**Chicken Marsala, 93**

**Rotisserie-Style Chicken, 95**

**Chicken Verde, 96**

**"Roasted" Turkey Legs, 97**

**Chicken Stir Fry, 99**

**Sweet and Smoky Chicken Thighs, 100**

**Easier Cheesy Chili Chicken, 101**

**Shredded Chicken Burrito Bowls, 103**

**Family-Style Chicken Breasts, 104**

**Cajun Turkey Tenderloin, 105**

**Creamy Chicken with Artichokes, 107**

**Orange Chicken, 108**

**Chicken with Broccoli Cheese Sauce, 109**

**Chicken Cacciatore, 111**

*Secret Message #4: The raw chicken in Christian's hands is the same chicken in the Rotisserie-Style Chicken photo on page 94.*

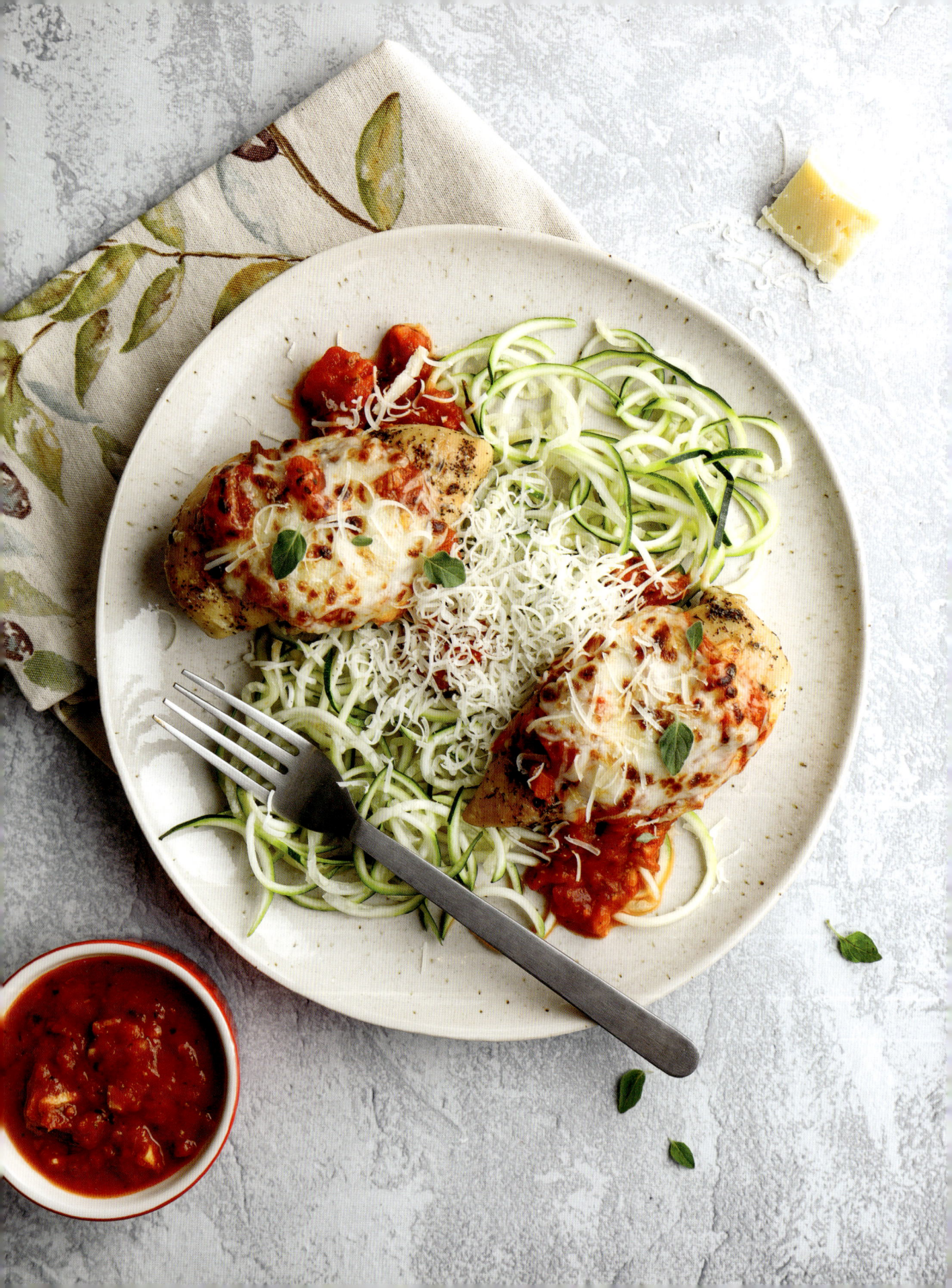

**Prep Time:** 5 min  |  **High Pressure:** 6 min  |  **Natural Release:** 5 min  |  **Serves:** 4

# Chicken Parmesan

We've always enjoyed Chicken Parmesan on low-carb by simply skipping the starchy breading. With the Instant Pot, we can always keep the chicken nice and moist, even without that breading to protect it.

## Ingredients

- 2 tablespoons olive oil
- 4 boneless, skinless chicken breasts
- 2 teaspoons minced garlic
- 2 cups chicken stock
- 1/4 teaspoon salt
- 1/4 teaspoon pepper
- 1 teaspoon Italian seasoning
- 1/3 cup no-sugar-added marinara sauce
- 1/4 cup grated or shredded Parmesan cheese
- 1/2 cup shredded mozzarella cheese

1. Heat olive oil in the Instant Pot on the SAUTÉ setting.
2. Add chicken breasts to the cooker and brown well on at least one side. Flip chicken and turn off cooker.
3. Add garlic to the chicken stock and pour in cooker, letting the chicken breasts sit directly in the liquid.
4. Season the tops of the chicken breasts with salt, pepper, and Italian seasoning.
5. Lock lid in place and seal pressure release vent. Set cooker to HIGH pressure for 6 minutes.
6. Let pressure release naturally for 5 minutes before opening vent to release any remaining pressure.
7. Remove chicken breasts from liquid and transfer to a sheet pan. Top each with an equal amount of the marinara sauce, then Parmesan cheese, then mozzarella cheese.
8. Place under broiler for 3–4 minutes or until cheese is bubbly and beginning to brown. Serve immediately.

### Instant Tips

For the best results, add enough chicken stock to bring the water level about 3/4 of the way up the chicken breasts. You want them mostly submerged to stay moist (by poaching) but with the tops exposed to keep the browned portion from washing away.

**Calories:** 330  |  **Fat:** 16g  |  **Protein:** 46.5g  |  **Total Carbs:** 3g  -  **Fiber:** 0g  =  **Net Carbs:** 3g

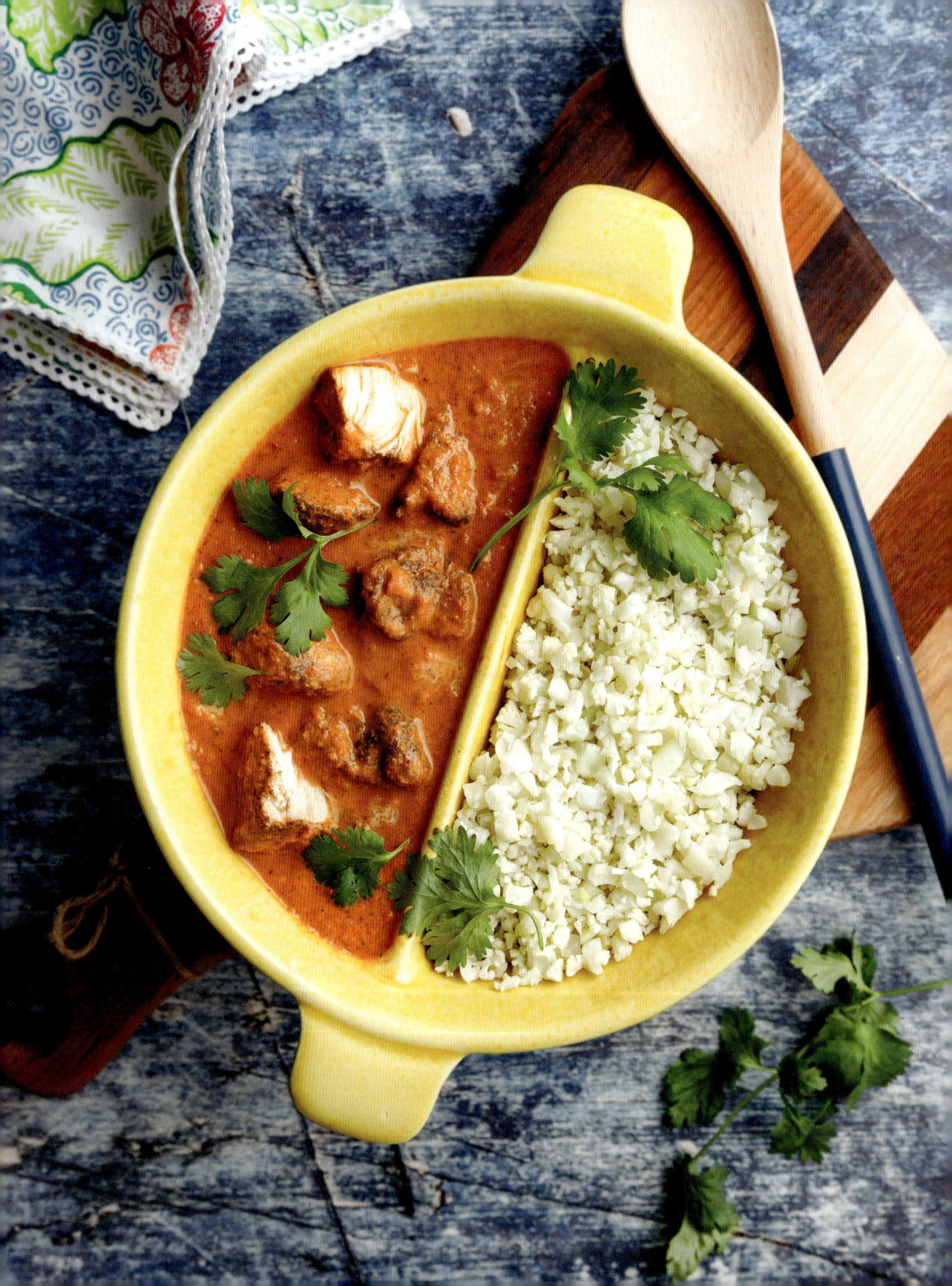

Prep Time: 15 min | High Pressure: 2 min | Quick Release | Serves: 4

# Indian Butter Chicken

In this recipe, chunks of boneless chicken breast are stewed in a buttery tomato sauce that is brimming with earthy Indian spices. For a full meal, serve alongside steamed cauliflower rice.

## Ingredients

3 tablespoons butter

1 tablespoon vegetable oil

1 1/2 pounds boneless, skinless chicken breast, chopped large

2 tablespoons garam masala

1 tablespoon minced garlic

1 tablespoon grated fresh ginger

1 (15-ounce) can diced tomatoes, with liquid

1/2 cup chopped yellow onion

1/4 cup chicken stock

2 teaspoons chili powder

2 teaspoons ground coriander

1 teaspoon ground cumin

3/4 teaspoon salt

1/2 teaspoon onion powder

1/2 cup heavy cream

Chopped fresh cilantro

1. Heat butter and vegetable oil in the Instant Pot on the SAUTÉ setting.

2. Toss chopped chicken breast in garam masala to thoroughly coat before adding to the cooker. Sauté until chicken begins to lightly brown.

3. Add garlic and ginger and sauté for 1 additional minute.

4. In a food processor or blender, blend together tomatoes, onion, chicken stock, chili powder, coriander, cumin, salt, and onion powder. Pour over chicken in the cooker.

5. Lock lid in place and seal pressure release vent. Set cooker to HIGH pressure for 2 minutes.

6. Carefully open vent to quickly release the pressure.

7. Set Instant Pot to SAUTÉ, add heavy cream, and bring up to a simmer. Let simmer 3 minutes or until slightly thickened.

8. Serve topped with plenty of chopped cilantro.

## Instant Tips

Garam masala is a dry spice blend often sold in the ethnic foods section but may also be found in the spice section.

Calories: 420 | Fat: 28.5g | Protein: 36.5g | Total Carbs: 8.5g - Fiber: 1.5g = Net Carbs: 7g

Prep Time: 10 min | High Pressure: 15 min | Natural Release: 5 min | Serves: 4

# Honey Mustard Chicken Drumsticks

Tender chicken legs are tossed in a tangy, semisweet mustard sauce in this family-favorite recipe. Guaranteed to make you ignore the napkin and lick your fingers clean instead.

## Ingredients

1 cup chicken stock
2 tablespoons Dijon mustard
3 pounds chicken legs
Salt and pepper
3 tablespoons mayonnaise
3 tablespoons yellow mustard
1 1/2 teaspoons sugar substitute
1/4 teaspoon garlic powder

## Special Equipment

Steam rack

1. Whisk chicken stock and Dijon mustard in Instant Pot until combined, then insert a steam rack.

2. Generously season chicken legs with salt and pepper before placing on the rack in the cooker.

3. Lock lid in place and seal pressure release vent. Set cooker to HIGH pressure for 15 minutes.

4. Let pressure release naturally for 5 minutes before opening vent to release any remaining pressure.

5. In a large mixing bowl, whisk together mayonnaise, yellow mustard, sugar substitute, and garlic powder.

6. Transfer cooked chicken legs to the mixing bowl and toss to evenly coat in the mustard sauce.

7. Transfer coated chicken legs to a sheet pan and place under broiler for 3 minutes or until drumsticks begin to brown. For the best texture, flip and broil again on the opposite side before serving.

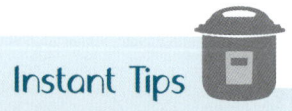

**Instant Tips**

This can also be made with only Dijon mustard in both the cooker and sauce for more of an "adult" flavor with a good kick of spice.

Calories: 670 | Fat: 28g | Protein: 96.5g | Total Carbs: 1g - Fiber: 0g = Net Carbs: 1g

Prep Time: 10 min | High Pressure: 5 min | Natural Release: 5 min | Serves: 4

# Chicken Marsala

Boneless, skinless chicken breasts are pressure cooked with marsala wine and baby bella mushrooms to make this simple variation on a classic dish. To lower the carbs, we simply do not dredge the chicken in flour before cooking.

## Ingredients

2 tablespoons olive oil

4 boneless, skinless chicken breasts

Salt and pepper

8 ounces baby bella mushrooms, quartered

2 shallots, diced

2 teaspoons minced garlic

1 teaspoon beef base

3/4 cup dry red wine

2 tablespoons butter

1. Heat olive oil in the Instant Pot on the SAUTÉ setting.

2. Generously season chicken breasts with salt and pepper before adding to the cooker and browning on at least one side.

3. Add the mushrooms, shallots, and garlic and move chicken breasts over top vegetables.

4. Whisk beef base into the wine before pouring into the cooker. Bring up to a simmer.

5. Lock lid in place and seal pressure release vent. Set cooker to HIGH pressure for 5 minutes.

6. Let pressure release naturally for 5 minutes before opening vent to release any remaining pressure.

7. Remove chicken breasts and set aside. Set cooker to SAUTÉ and bring sauce back up to a simmer, cooking until sauce has reduced by about 1/2.

8. Turn off cooker and stir in butter before seasoning sauce with salt and pepper to taste. Return chicken to the sauce to warm through before serving.

### Instant Tips

Marsala cooking wine is extremely sweet, so we just use a dry cabernet. We also like to add a splash of heavy cream to the sauce after cooking.

Calories: 375 | Fat: 17.5g | Protein: 42.5g | Total Carbs: 5.5g - Fiber: 0.5g = Net Carbs: 5g

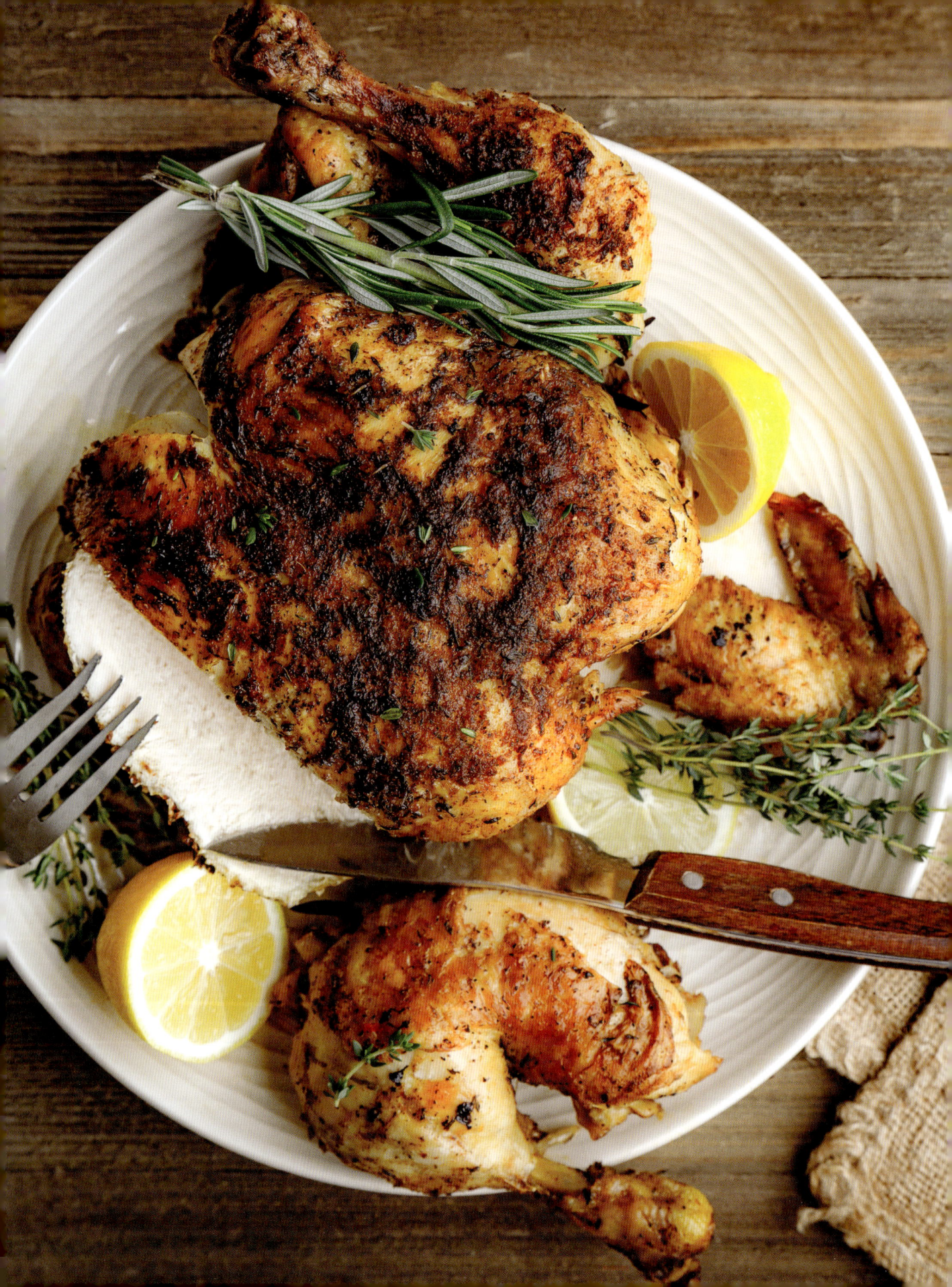

Prep Time: 10 min | High Pressure: 30 min | Natural Release: 15 min | Serves: 6

# Rotisserie-Style Chicken

Our local deli never turned out a chicken quite as juicy as this, as it falls apart every time, but we don't view that as a bad thing since it saves us from having to do so much carving.

## Ingredients

1 (5-pound) whole chicken, giblets removed

Juice of 1/2 lemon

2 teaspoons paprika

1 1/2 teaspoons salt

1 1/2 teaspoons dried thyme

1 teaspoon dried rosemary

1 teaspoon pepper

1/2 teaspoon garlic powder

1/2 teaspoon onion powder

3 tablespoons olive oil

1/2 cup chicken stock

1/2 lemon, cut into wedges

1 sprig fresh rosemary, optional

1 sprig fresh thyme, optional

1. Drizzle chicken with lemon juice before thoroughly coating with all spices.
2. Heat olive oil in the Instant Pot on the SAUTÉ setting.
3. Carefully place chicken, breast-side down, in the cooker and brown well, about 7 minutes.
4. Flip chicken and brown on opposite side for 6 minutes. Turn off cooker.
5. If there is room in your cooker, place chicken on a steam rack before lowering back into the cooker. This will keep the bottom of the chicken crispier but is entirely optional.
6. Pour chicken stock into cooker and arrange lemon wedges and fresh herbs around the chicken. Fresh herbs are also optional but infuse more flavor.
7. Lock lid in place and seal pressure release vent. Set cooker to HIGH pressure for 30 minutes.
8. Let pressure release naturally for 15 minutes before opening vent to release any remaining pressure.
9. For the crispiest skin, place oven rack in center position and broil chicken for 5 minutes or until skin is well browned. Let rest 10 minutes before carving to serve.

### Instant Tips

For a 4-pound chicken, reduce cooking time to 26 minutes. For a 6-pound chicken, increase cooking time to 36 minutes, but be aware that a 6-pound chicken is a very tight fit in a 6 quart cooker.

Calories: 315 | Fat: 20.5g | Protein: 17g | Total Carbs: 3g - Fiber: 1g = Net Carbs: 2g

Prep Time: 15 min | High Pressure: 15 min | Natural Release: 10 min | Serves: 4

# Chicken Verde

Bone-in chicken thighs are cooked in green salsa in this simple entrée you can make any day of the week. For a full meal, serve alongside plenty of cauliflower rice.

## Ingredients

2 tablespoons olive oil
1/2 green bell pepper, chopped
1/2 cup diced yellow onion
1 tablespoon minced garlic
3/4 cup salsa verde
1/4 cup chicken stock
1/4 cup chopped fresh cilantro
1 teaspoon sugar substitute
3/4 teaspoon ground cumin
2 pounds bone-in chicken thighs, skin removed
Salt and pepper
Sour cream, to top

1. Heat olive oil in the Instant Pot on the SAUTÉ setting.
2. Add bell pepper, onion, and garlic and sauté 3 minutes or until onion begins to turn translucent.
3. Stir in salsa, chicken stock, cilantro, sugar substitute, and cumin.
4. Generously season chicken thighs with salt and pepper before adding to the sauce in the cooker.
5. Lock lid in place and seal pressure release vent. Set cooker to HIGH pressure for 15 minutes.
6. Let pressure release naturally for 10 minutes before opening vent to release any remaining pressure.
7. Serve chicken topped with the sauce and a dollop of sour cream.

**Instant Tips**

For a bit more spice, we like to add a seeded and diced jalapeño to this soup before pressure cooking.

Calories: 345 | Fat: 21g | Protein: 36.5g | Total Carbs: 5.5g  -  Fiber: 0.5g  =  Net Carbs: 5g

Prep Time: 10 min | High Pressure: 20 min | Natural Release: 10 min | Serves: 4

# "Roasted" Turkey Legs

A staple of county fairs and Disney World, turkey legs are now sold in most grocery stores. Oven roasting them can take well over an hour to get the same tender results you can get in only 30 minutes of pressure cooking and natural release.

## Ingredients

4 turkey legs
¼ cup chicken stock
¼ cup soy sauce
2 tablespoons butter, melted
1 tablespoon chopped fresh sage
½ teaspoon dried rosemary
½ teaspoon salt
½ teaspoon pepper
¼ teaspoon garlic powder

## Special Equipment

Steam rack

1. Insert steam rack into the Instant Pot and top with turkey legs.
2. Whisk together chicken stock, soy sauce, and butter and pour over turkey legs, moving the legs as needed to ensure each one gets a light coating of the liquid.
3. Season the turkey legs with sage, rosemary, salt, pepper, and garlic powder.
4. Lock lid in place and seal pressure release vent. Set cooker to HIGH pressure for 20 minutes.
5. Let pressure release naturally for 10 minutes before opening vent to release any remaining pressure.
6. Transfer the cooked turkey legs to a sheet pan and drizzle with a small amount of the liquid from the cooker.
7. Place under broiler for 4 minutes on each side or until skin has browned. Serve drizzled with additional liquid from the cooker.

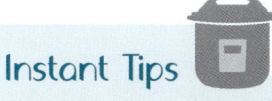

**Instant Tips**

For even more flavor, let the liquid in the cooker reduce on the SAUTÉ setting before drizzling over the legs and broiling.

Calories: 480 | Fat: 24g | Protein: 61g | Total Carbs: 0.5g - Fiber: 0g = Net Carbs: 0.5g

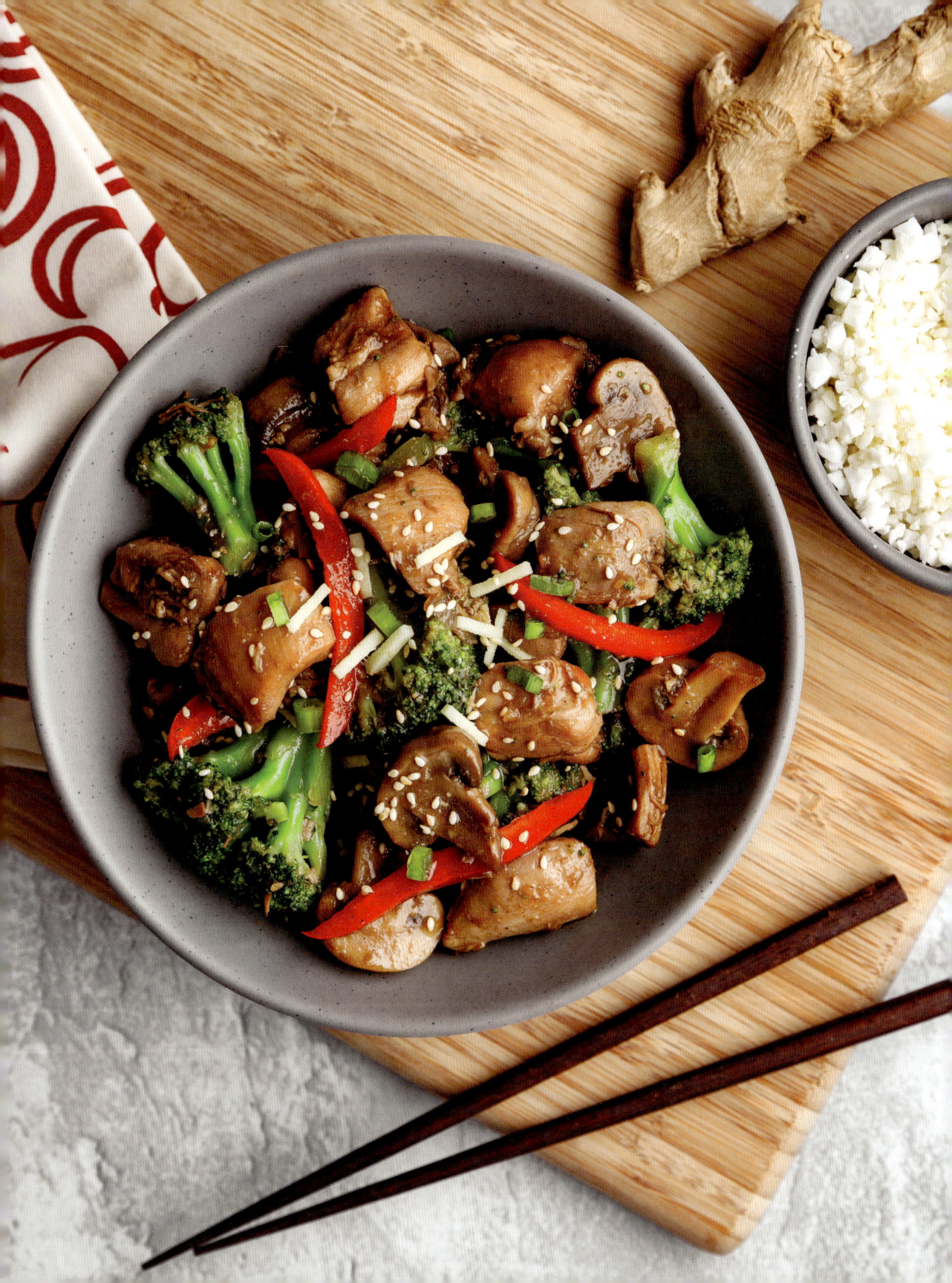

Prep Time: 15 min | High Pressure: 5 min | Quick Release | Serves: 4

# Chicken Stir Fry

While a stir fry can be cooked quickly on the stove, cooking this stir fry under pressure ensures tender chopped chicken thighs and a marriage of flavors that is hard to reproduce any other way.

## Ingredients

1 tablespoon vegetable oil

1 1/2 pounds boneless, skinless chicken thighs, chopped into 1-inch pieces

8 ounces button mushrooms, halved

1/2 cup sliced red onion

2 teaspoons minced garlic

2 teaspoons grated fresh ginger

1 teaspoon Chinese five-spice powder

2 teaspoons sugar substitute

1/4 teaspoon onion powder

1/4 cup soy sauce

1 tablespoon rice wine vinegar

12 ounces frozen broccoli florets

1/2 red bell pepper, thinly sliced

1 tablespoon sesame oil

1. Heat vegetable oil in the Instant Pot on the SAUTÉ setting.

2. Add chicken thighs to the cooker and sauté until they begin to lightly brown.

3. Add the mushrooms, onion, and garlic and sauté 2 minutes before stirring in ginger, five-spice powder, sugar substitute, and onion powder until everything is coated in the spices.

4. Stir in soy sauce and rice wine vinegar.

5. Lock lid in place and seal pressure release vent. Set cooker to HIGH pressure for 5 minutes.

6. Carefully open vent to quickly release the pressure.

7. Set Instant Pot to SAUTÉ, add frozen broccoli and red bell pepper, and bring up to a simmer. Let cook until broccoli is tender and liquid has reduced by at least 1/3.

8. Stir in sesame oil before serving. For the brightest flavor, stir an additional splash of rice wine vinegar and an additional teaspoon of fresh ginger in right before serving to wake up the flavors.

### Instant Tips

The fresh ginger really adds a brightness to this recipe that you can't get from a spice jar; however, 1/4 teaspoon of ground ginger can be used in its place in a pinch.

Calories: 340 | Fat: 19g | Protein: 36g | Total Carbs: 9.5g - Fiber: 3g = Net Carbs: 6.5g

Prep Time: 10 min | High Pressure: 10 min | Natural Release: 10 min | Serves: 4

# Sweet and Smoky Chicken Thighs

Bone-in chicken thighs are rubbed with smoked paprika and a hint of sugar substitute for sweetness in this simple recipe, with all of the flavors of barbecue chicken without the extra carbs found in tomato-based sauces.

## Ingredients

2 tablespoons vegetable oil, divided

2 pounds bone-in chicken thighs, skin removed

1 tablespoon smoked paprika

1 teaspoon sugar substitute

¾ teaspoon salt

½ teaspoon garlic powder

¼ teaspoon onion powder

¼ teaspoon pepper

1 cup chicken stock

1. Pour 1 tablespoon of the vegetable oil into a large mixing bowl. Add chicken thighs, smoked paprika, sugar substitute, salt, garlic powder, onion powder, and pepper and toss to fully coat chicken.

2. Heat the remaining tablespoon of vegetable oil in the Instant Pot on the SAUTÉ setting.

3. Brown the chicken thighs on at least one side before positioning browned side up.

4. Pour chicken stock into the cooker.

5. Lock lid in place and seal pressure release vent. Set cooker to HIGH pressure for 10 minutes.

6. Let pressure release naturally for 10 minutes before opening vent to release any remaining pressure. Remove chicken from liquid and serve immediately.

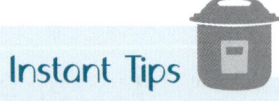

### Instant Tips

You can make these with boneless, skinless chicken thighs, reducing the time under pressure to 8 minutes.

Calories: 330 | Fat: 21g | Protein: 36.5g | Total Carbs: 1.5g - Fiber: 0.5g = Net Carbs: 1g

Prep Time: 15 min | High Pressure: 8 min | Natural Release: 5 min | Serves: 4

# Easier Cheesy Chili Chicken

Based on one of our most popular recipes of all time, this recipe is made even easier and far faster, thanks to the Instant Pot. Chicken breasts are heavily seasoned with a mixture of earthy chili spices before being topped with red onion, tomato, and Cheddar-Jack cheese.

## Ingredients

1 cup chicken stock

4 boneless, skinless chicken breasts

2 tablespoons extra-virgin olive oil

2 tablespoons chopped cilantro

1 tablespoon chili powder

2 teaspoons ground cumin

3/4 teaspoon salt

1/2 teaspoon pepper

1/4 teaspoon garlic powder

1/8 teaspoon ground cayenne pepper

1/4 cup thinly sliced green bell pepper

2 tablespoons minced red onion

1/4 cup diced tomato

3/4 cup shredded Cheddar-Jack cheese

## Special Equipment

Steam rack

1. Pour chicken stock into the Instant Pot and place a steam rack over top.

2. In a mixing bowl, toss chicken breasts with olive oil, cilantro, chili powder, cumin, salt, pepper, garlic powder, and cayenne pepper until well coated.

3. Place the coated chicken breasts on the steam rack in the cooker and top each with an equal amount of the green bell pepper and red onion.

4. Lock lid in place and seal pressure release vent. Set cooker to HIGH pressure for 8 minutes.

5. Let pressure release naturally for 5 minutes before opening vent to release any remaining pressure.

6. Transfer chicken breasts to a sheet pan. Top each with an equal amount of the diced tomato and Cheddar-Jack cheese.

7. Place under broiler for 2 minutes or until cheese is bubbly hot. Serve immediately.

### Instant Tips

You can make these chicken breasts using just the delicious spice rub and omitting the green bell pepper, red onion, tomato, and even the Cheddar-Jack cheese. This also allows you to skip the broiling step.

Calories: 355 | Fat: 19g | Protein: 45g | Total Carbs: 3g - Fiber: 1g = Net Carbs: 2g

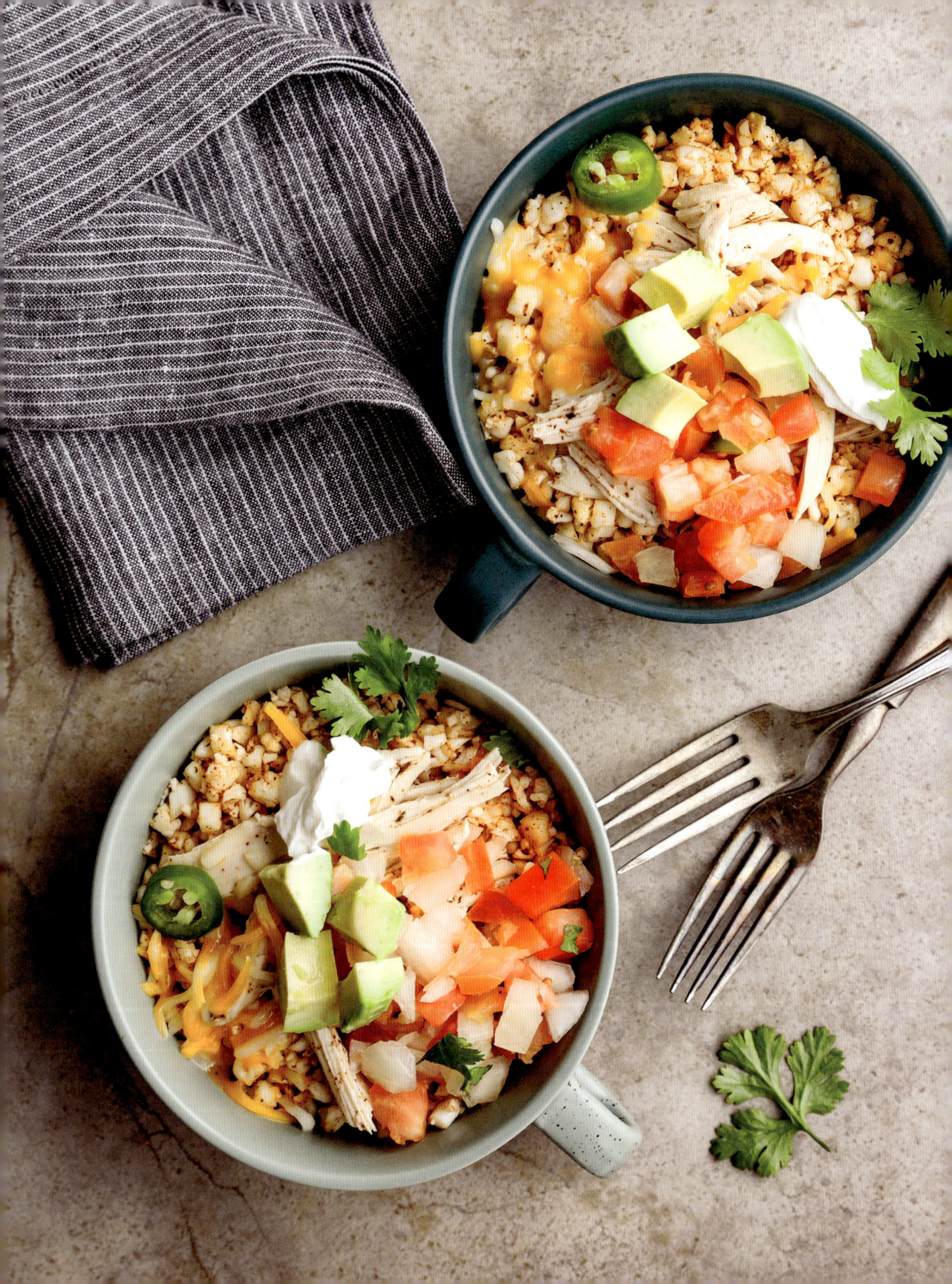

Prep Time: 25 min | High Pressure: 20 min | Natural Release: 5 min | Serves: 4

# Shredded Chicken Burrito Bowls

Chicken breasts are cooked in salsa before being shredded to fill out these cauliflower-rice bowls. We like to then top the bowls with Colby-Jack cheese, fresh pico de gallo, avocado, and sour cream, but you can choose your own favorite taco/burrito toppings!

## Ingredients

3 boneless, skinless chicken breasts
1/2 cup chicken stock
1/2 cup jarred salsa
Juice of 1/2 lime
1 teaspoon chili powder
1/2 teaspoon salt
1/2 teaspoon pepper

### Seasoned Rice

2 tablespoons olive oil
12 ounces grated cauliflower (1 small head)
2 teaspoons minced garlic
2 teaspoons chili powder
1/2 teaspoon ground cumin
Salt and pepper

### Burrito Bowls

1 cup Colby-Jack cheese
1/2 cup fresh pico de gallo
1 avocado, chopped
1/4 cup sour cream

1. In the Instant Pot, toss chicken breasts in chicken stock, salsa, lime juice, chili powder, salt, and pepper.

2. Lock lid in place and seal pressure release vent. Set cooker to HIGH pressure for 20 minutes.

3. Let pressure release naturally for 5 minutes before opening vent to release any remaining pressure.

4. Meanwhile, make the Seasoned Rice by heating olive oil in a large skillet over medium-high heat.

5. Add the cauliflower, garlic, chili powder, and cumin to the skillet and sauté for 5 minutes or until cauliflower begins to brown. Season with salt and pepper to taste, cover skillet, and remove from heat until ready to prepare the bowls.

6. Using two forks, shred the cooked chicken into the liquid in the Instant Pot.

7. Assemble the Burrito Bowls by filling 4 serving bowls with the cauliflower rice and using a slotted spoon to top with shredded chicken from the cooker.

8. Top each bowl with an equal amount of the Colby-Jack cheese, pico de gallo, avocado, and sour cream before serving.

### Instant Tips

This recipe makes 4 big bowls, but for even more leftovers, you can cook a fourth chicken breast in the same amount of liquid.

Calories: 460 | Fat: 29g | Protein: 38.5g | Total Carbs: 15g - Fiber: 6g = Net Carbs: 9g

Prep Time: 5 min | High Pressure: 12 min | Natural Release: 10 min | Serves: 4

# Family-Style Chicken Breasts

Seasoned with mostly pantry staples, try serving these bone-in chicken breasts alongside a big bowl of mixed salad or your favorite steamed vegetables.

## Ingredients

1 cup chicken stock

Juice of 1/2 lemon

2 tablespoons butter, melted

4 bone-in chicken breasts, skin removed

1 1/2 teaspoons paprika

3/4 teaspoon salt

1/2 teaspoon dried thyme

1/2 teaspoon dried rosemary

1/2 teaspoon poultry seasoning

1/2 teaspoon pepper

1. Pour chicken stock and lemon juice into Instant Pot.
2. Drizzle melted butter over chicken breasts.
3. Combine all spices and sprinkle over chicken breasts until heavily seasoned (use all of the spice mixture).
4. Place chicken breasts in cooker, breast-side up, stacking them as necessary.
5. Lock lid in place and seal pressure release vent. Set cooker to HIGH pressure for 12 minutes.
6. Let pressure release naturally for 10 minutes before opening vent to release any remaining pressure. Remove chicken from liquid and serve immediately.

### Instant Tips

You can make this chicken with the skin, but you will want to place the chicken under the broiler after pressure cooking to crisp up the skin.

Calories: 255 | Fat: 11g | Protein: 40.5g | Total Carbs: 1g - Fiber: 0g = Net Carbs: 1g

Prep Time: 10 min | High Pressure: 20 min | Natural Release: 10 min | Serves: 4

# Cajun Turkey Tenderloin

Turkey tenderloin is a simple way to enjoy turkey without cooking an entire bird or breast. In this recipe, we rub the tenderloin with Cajun spices that also help season a creamy pan gravy made in only a few minutes after pressure cooking.

## Ingredients

- 1 turkey tenderloin
- 2 teaspoons paprika
- 1 teaspoon dried thyme
- 1 teaspoon salt
- 3/4 teaspoon pepper
- 1/2 teaspoon garlic powder
- 1/2 teaspoon onion powder
- 1/2 teaspoon cayenne pepper
- 2 tablespoons vegetable oil
- 1/2 cup chicken stock
- 1/2 cup heavy cream

1. Rub the turkey tenderloin with all spices.
2. Heat vegetable oil in the Instant Pot on the SAUTÉ setting.
3. Place the seasoned turkey tenderloin in the cooker and brown on at least two sides before pouring in chicken stock.
4. Lock lid in place and seal pressure release vent. Set cooker to HIGH pressure for 20 minutes.
5. Let pressure release naturally for 10 minutes before opening vent to release any remaining pressure.
6. Transfer turkey tenderloin to a plate and cover with aluminum foil to rest.
7. Set cooker to SAUTÉ, stir in heavy cream, and bring up to a simmer. Let simmer until reduced by about 1/3.
8. Carve turkey tenderloin and serve drizzled with gravy from the cooker.

### Instant Tips

This can also be made with 4 to 6 boneless, skinless chicken breasts, reducing the pressure cooking time to 6 minutes.

Calories: 300 | Fat: 20.5g | Protein: 32g | Total Carbs: 1.5g - Fiber: 0g = Net Carbs: 1.5g

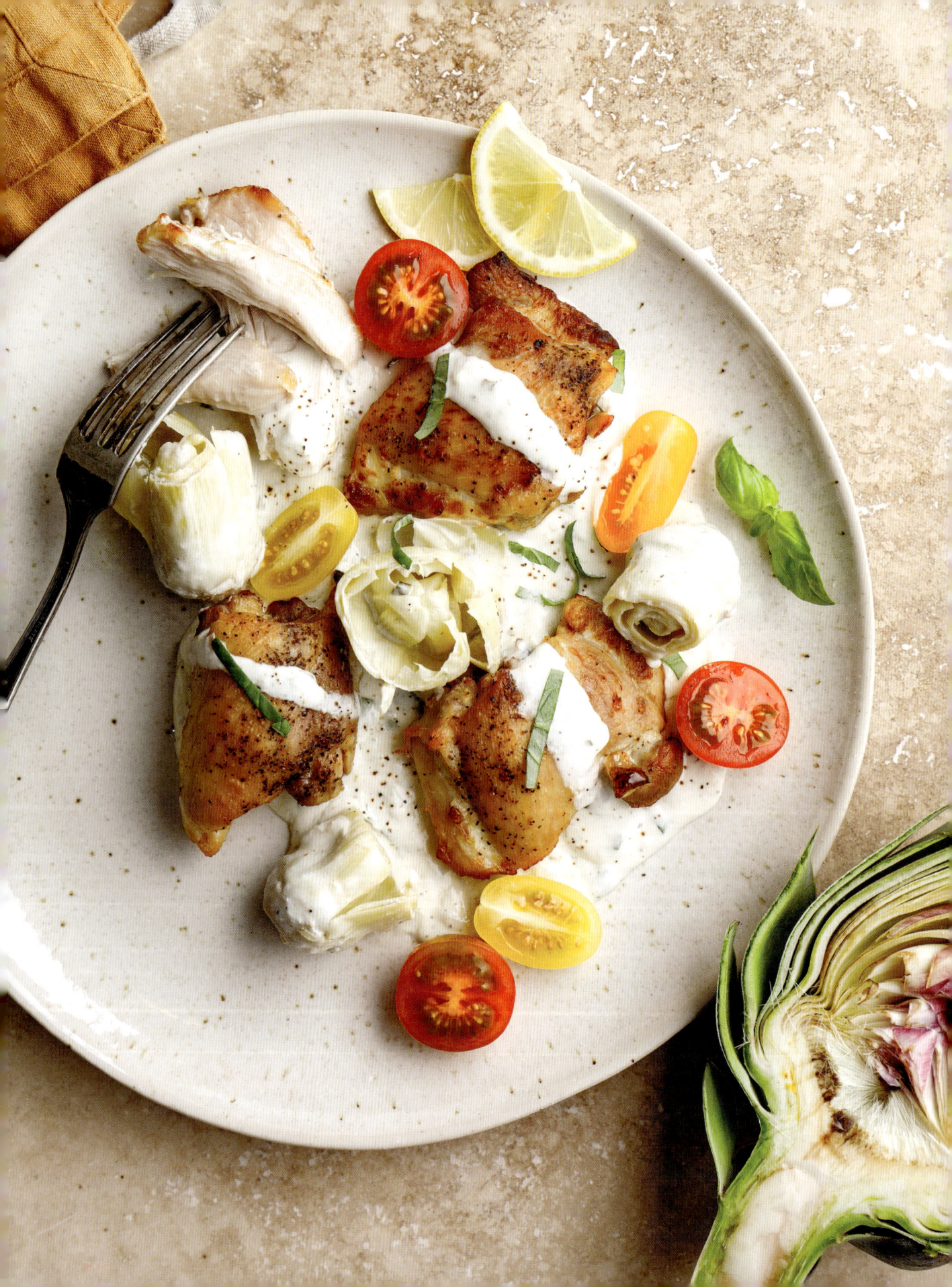

Prep Time: 20 min | High Pressure: 10 min | Natural Release: 10 min | Serves: 4

# Creamy Chicken with Artichokes

Boneless chicken thighs are cooked with fresh basil before being tossed in a creamy sauce made from herbed cream cheese. The artichoke hearts and grape tomatoes are added only after pressure cooking to keep them fresh and vibrant.

## Ingredients

- 2 tablespoons olive oil
- 2 pounds boneless, skinless chicken thighs
- Salt and pepper
- 1 tablespoon minced garlic
- 1/2 cup diced red onion
- 1/2 cup chicken stock
- 1/4 cup chopped fresh basil, divided
- 1 tablespoon lemon juice
- 1 (14-ounce) can artichoke hearts, drained
- 4 ounces herbed cream cheese
- 1 cup grape tomatoes, halved

1. Heat olive oil in the Instant Pot on the SAUTÉ setting.
2. Generously season chicken thighs with salt and pepper before adding to the cooker and browning on at least one side.
3. Add the garlic and onion to the cooker and sauté for 1 minute before adding chicken stock, 1/2 of the fresh basil, and lemon juice.
4. Lock lid in place and seal pressure release vent. Set cooker to HIGH pressure for 10 minutes.
5. Let pressure release naturally for 10 minutes before opening vent to release any remaining pressure.
6. Set aside chicken thighs and drain 1/2 of the liquid from the cooker.
7. Set cooker to SAUTÉ and add artichoke hearts. Bring up to a simmer for 3 minutes.
8. Turn off heat and stir in cream cheese until melted into the sauce. Stir in grape tomatoes and the remaining 1/2 of the basil before seasoning with salt and pepper to taste and serving over the chicken thighs.

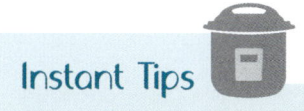

**Instant Tips**

We also like to top this with a little bit of fresh lemon zest and shredded Parmesan cheese.

Calories: 510 | Fat: 33g | Protein: 48g | Total Carbs: 8g - Fiber: 2g = Net Carbs: 6g

Prep Time: 10 min | High Pressure: 3 min | Quick Release | Serves: 4

# Orange Chicken

This Asian-inspired dish has chunks of chicken breasts in a sweet and somewhat spicy sauce with a kick of orange zest.

## Ingredients

- 1 tablespoon sesame oil
- 4 boneless, skinless chicken breasts, cut into 1 1/2-inch chunks
- 1 teaspoon minced garlic
- 1/4 cup soy sauce
- 1 tablespoon cider vinegar
- 1 tablespoon orange zest
- 1 tablespoon sugar substitute
- 1/4 teaspoon crushed red pepper flakes
- 1 tablespoon butter
- 1/4 cup sliced scallions

1. Heat sesame oil in the Instant Pot on the SAUTÉ setting.
2. Add chicken to the cooker and sauté until it begins to lightly brown.
3. Add garlic and sauté for 1 additional minute.
4. Stir in soy sauce, cider vinegar, orange zest, sugar substitute, and red pepper flakes.
5. Lock lid in place and seal pressure release vent. Set cooker to HIGH pressure for 3 minutes.
6. Carefully open vent to quickly release the pressure.
7. Set Instant Pot to SAUTÉ and cook until the sauce has slightly thickened and begins to better coat the chicken.
8. Turn off cooker and stir in butter before serving topped with sliced scallions.

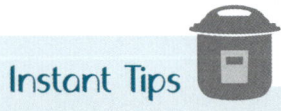

### Instant Tips

We like to add 2 chopped zucchini and 1/2 cup of diced bell peppers to this after pressure cooking (as we are thickening the sauce) to make a full meal.

Calories: 260 | Fat: 10.5g | Protein: 41.5g | Total Carbs: 2g - Fiber: 0g = Net Carbs: 2g

Prep Time: 10 min | High Pressure: 6 min | Quick Release | Serves: 4

# Chicken with Broccoli Cheese Sauce

There's nothing more family-friendly than chicken and broccoli smothered in a creamy cheese sauce. Adding a touch of Dijon mustard in the last step makes the sauce even more rich and flavorful.

## Ingredients

4 boneless, skinless chicken breasts

Salt and pepper

Garlic powder

2 cups broccoli florets

½ cup diced yellow onion

½ cup chicken stock

½ cup heavy cream

1 cup shredded sharp Cheddar cheese

1 tablespoon Dijon mustard

1. Generously season chicken breasts with salt, pepper, and garlic powder and place in Instant Pot.
2. Top chicken breasts with broccoli and onion before pouring in chicken stock.
3. Lock lid in place and seal pressure release vent. Set cooker to HIGH pressure for 6 minutes.
4. Carefully open vent to quickly release the pressure.
5. Set aside chicken breasts and cover with aluminum foil.
6. Set Instant Pot to SAUTÉ, add heavy cream, and bring up to a simmer. Let simmer until liquid has reduced by about ⅓. Much of the broccoli will melt into the sauce.
7. Turn cooker off and stir in Cheddar cheese and Dijon mustard before seasoning sauce with salt and pepper to taste.
8. Return the chicken to the sauce before serving.

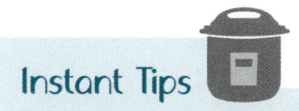

**Instant Tips**

For even more flavor, brown the chicken breasts in 1 tablespoon of vegetable oil and 1 tablespoon of butter before pressure cooking.

Calories: 440 | Fat: 26g | Protein: 47g | Total Carbs: 5g - Fiber: 1g = Net Carbs: 4g

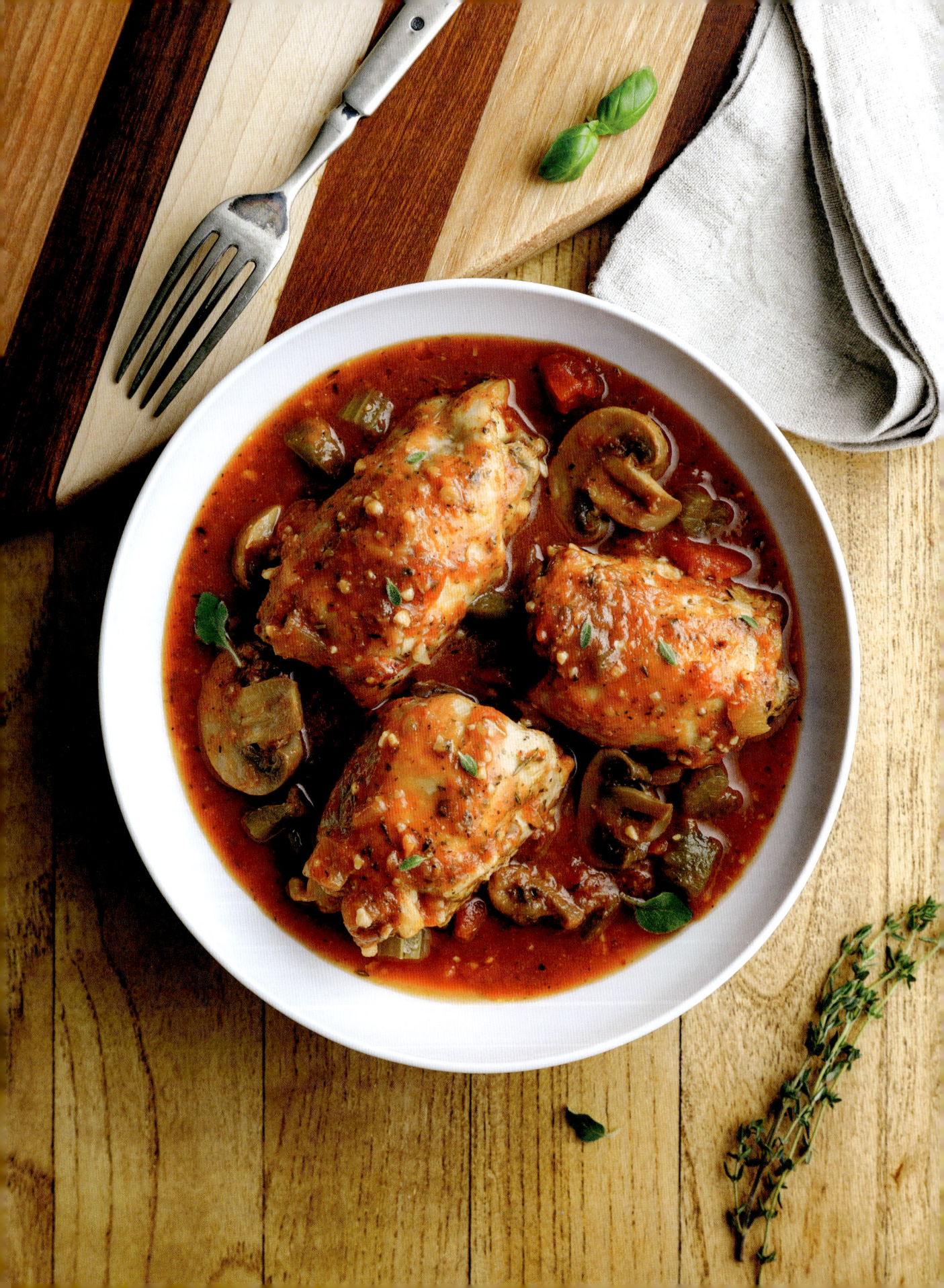

Prep Time: 15 min | High Pressure: 15 min | Natural Release: 10 min | Serves: 4

# Chicken Cacciatore

Cacciatore is a classic Italian dish that is usually stewed all day, but with this recipe, you can have a comforting meal on the table in only about an hour. To round out the dinner, we like to serve this with either spiralized zucchini noodles or cauliflower rice.

## Ingredients

- 2 tablespoons olive oil
- 8 ounces button mushrooms, halved
- ½ cup chopped celery
- ½ cup chopped green bell pepper
- ½ cup sliced red onion
- 1 tablespoon minced garlic
- 1 (15-ounce) can diced tomatoes, with liquid
- ¼ cup chicken stock
- 1 tablespoon balsamic vinegar
- 2 teaspoons Italian seasoning
- ¾ teaspoon salt
- ½ teaspoon pepper
- ¼ teaspoon crushed red pepper flakes
- 2 pounds bone-in chicken thighs, skin removed
- 2 tablespoons tomato paste
- 1 tablespoon butter

1. Heat olive oil in the Instant Pot on the SAUTÉ setting.
2. Add mushrooms, celery, bell pepper, onion, and garlic and sauté for 3 minutes or until onion begins to turn translucent.
3. Stir in tomatoes, chicken stock, balsamic vinegar, Italian seasoning, salt, pepper, and crushed red pepper flakes.
4. Add chicken and press down to partially submerge in the sauce.
5. Lock lid in place and seal pressure release vent. Set cooker to HIGH pressure for 15 minutes.
6. Let pressure release naturally for 10 minutes before opening vent to release any remaining pressure.
7. Set aside chicken thighs and stir tomato paste and butter into the sauce. Serve chicken topped with plenty of sauce and vegetables.

### Instant Tips

We like to brighten this up by serving it topped with a bit of fresh lemon zest and chopped flat-leaf parsley.

---

Calories: 405 | Fat: 24g | Protein: 39.5g | Total Carbs: 12g - Fiber: 3g = Net Carbs: 9g

*Chapter 5*

# Meats

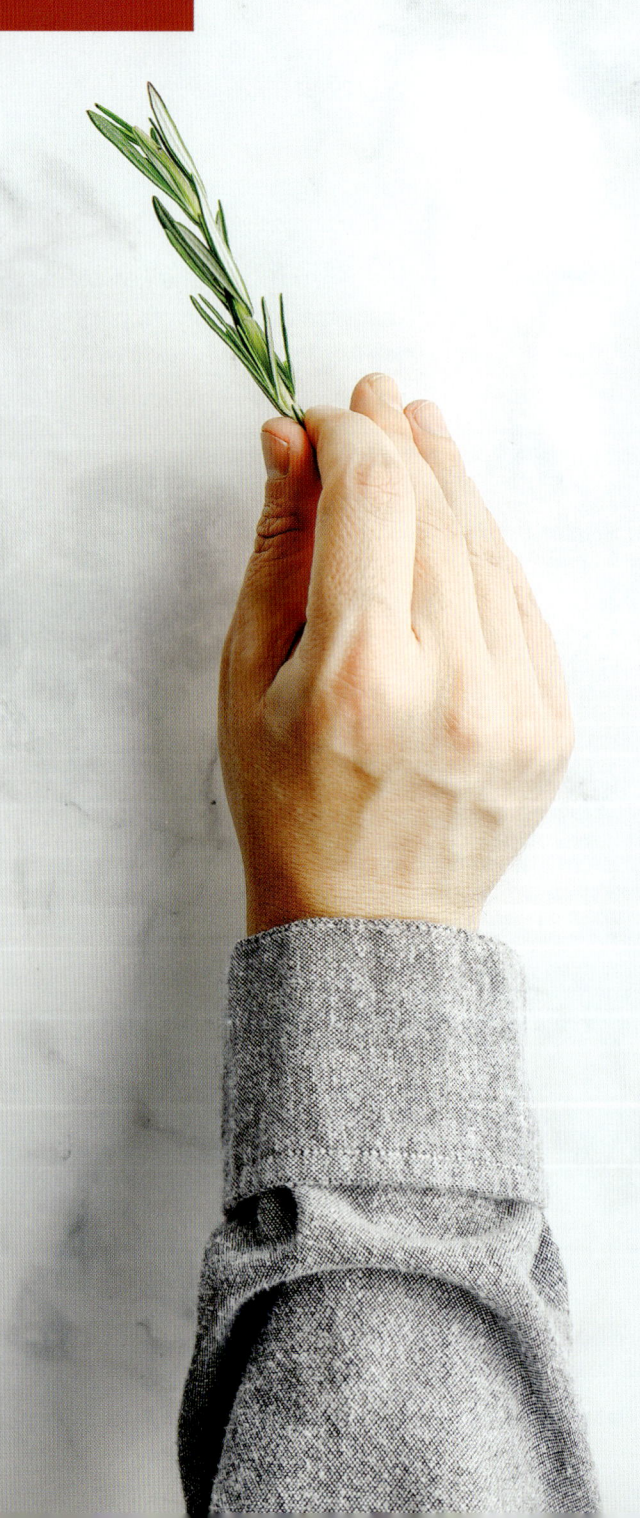

## recipes in this chapter...

**Instant Pot Roast**, 115

**Baby Back Ribs**, 117

**Jamaican Jerk Pork Shoulder**, 118

**Barbacoa Beef**, 119

**Bratwurst with Honey Mustard Kraut**, 121

**Beef Paprikash**, 122

**Greek Lamb Roast**, 123

**Barbecue Pulled Pork**, 125

**Sweet Onion Brisket**, 126

**Balsamic Braised Short Ribs**, 127

**Beef Stroganoff**, 129

**Tequila Pork Tenderloin**, 131

**Italian Sausage with Peppers and Kale**, 132

**Red Wine Braised Beef**, 133

**Mongolian Beef**, 135

**Boneless Ribs with Sweet Chili Sauce**, 136

**Pork Carnitas**, 137

**Corned Beef and Cabbage**, 139

Secret Message #5: We used white tequila (which looks like water) to make the Tequila Pork Tenderloin, so we had to then buy yellow tequila just to put a shot of it in the photograph!

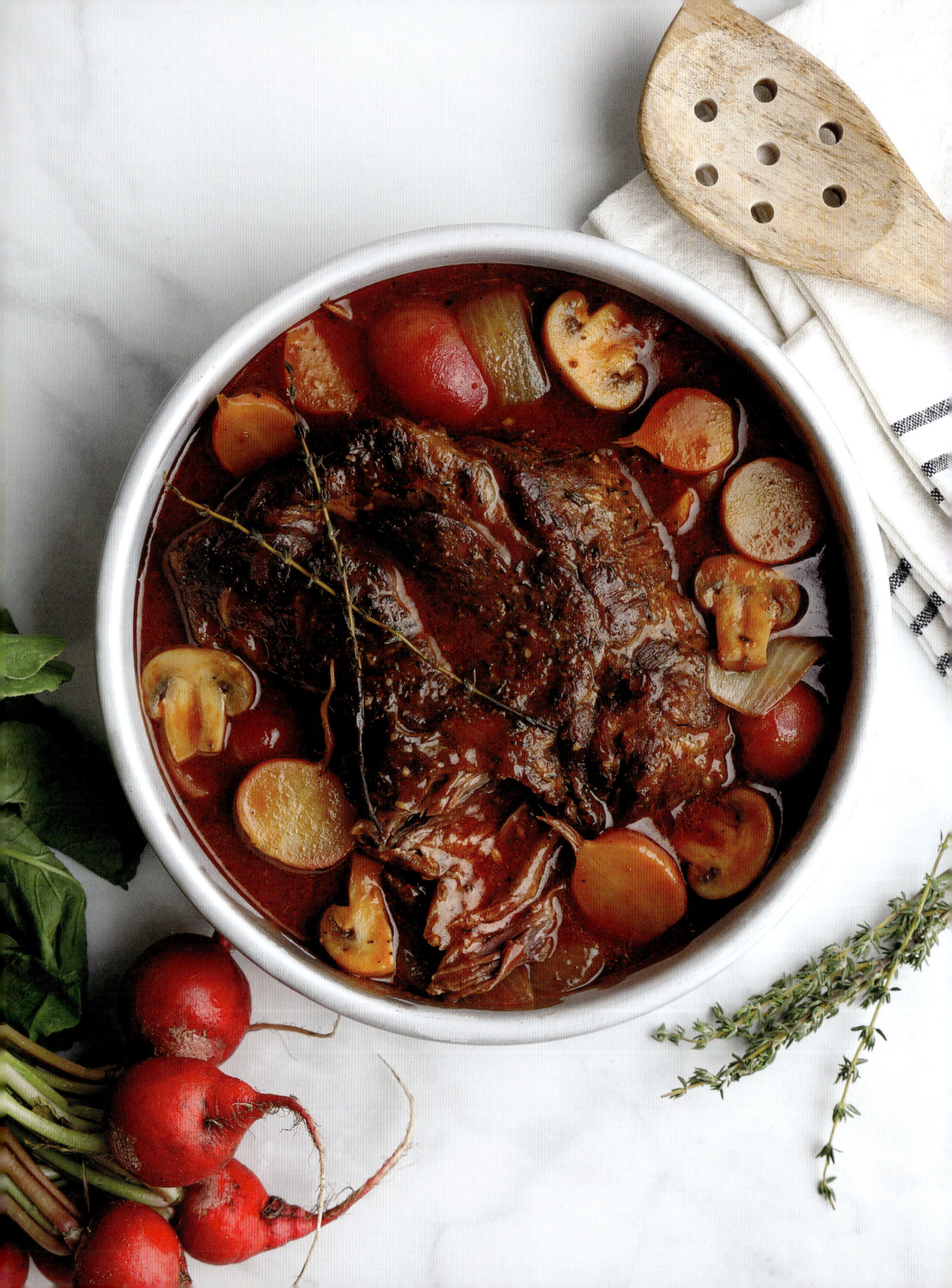

**Prep Time: 10 min | High Pressure: 75 min | Natural Release: 15 min | Serves: 6**

# Instant Pot Roast

If there is one reason to own an Instant Pot, that reason is… Pot Roast! There's no quicker way to get these incredibly tender results. But what makes this pot roast recipe so special is radishes, a sadly underused vegetable. Radishes are extremely low in carbohydrates with only around 2g of net carbs in an entire cup, yet they cook up almost exactly like a high-carb potato when boiled.

## Ingredients

2 tablespoons vegetable oil
1 (2.5 to 3.5-pound) chuck roast
Salt and pepper
1 cup beef stock
1 tablespoon minced garlic
2 sprigs fresh thyme
2 bay leaves
½ teaspoon dried thyme
½ teaspoon onion powder
1 small yellow onion, cut into wedges
8 ounces button mushrooms, halved
2 cups radishes, halved
2 tablespoons tomato paste
2 tablespoons butter

1. Heat vegetable oil in the Instant Pot on the SAUTÉ setting.

2. Generously season roast with salt and pepper on both sides. For larger roasts that are over 3 pounds, cut in half for the most tender results.

3. Add the seasoned roast to the cooker and brown well on both sides.

4. Add the beef stock, garlic, fresh thyme, bay leaves, dried thyme, and onion powder to the cooker.

5. Lock lid in place and seal pressure release vent. Set cooker to HIGH pressure for 75 minutes.

6. Let pressure release naturally for 15 minutes before opening vent to release any remaining pressure. Transfer roast to a plate and cover with aluminum foil.

7. Set cooker to SAUTÉ and add onion, mushrooms, and radishes. Let simmer 10 minutes or until radishes are tender.

8. Turn off cooker, stir in tomato paste and butter, and generously season pan gravy with salt and pepper to taste. Return roast to the pan gravy before pulling apart to serve.

### Instant Tips

When seasoning the pan gravy with salt and pepper, we also like to add a pinch or two of sugar substitute to add another dimension to the flavor. It also balances out a slight bitterness that the radishes add.

---

**Calories: 575 | Fat: 43.5g | Protein: 38g | Total Carbs: 6g  -  Fiber: 1.5g  =  Net Carbs: 4.5g**

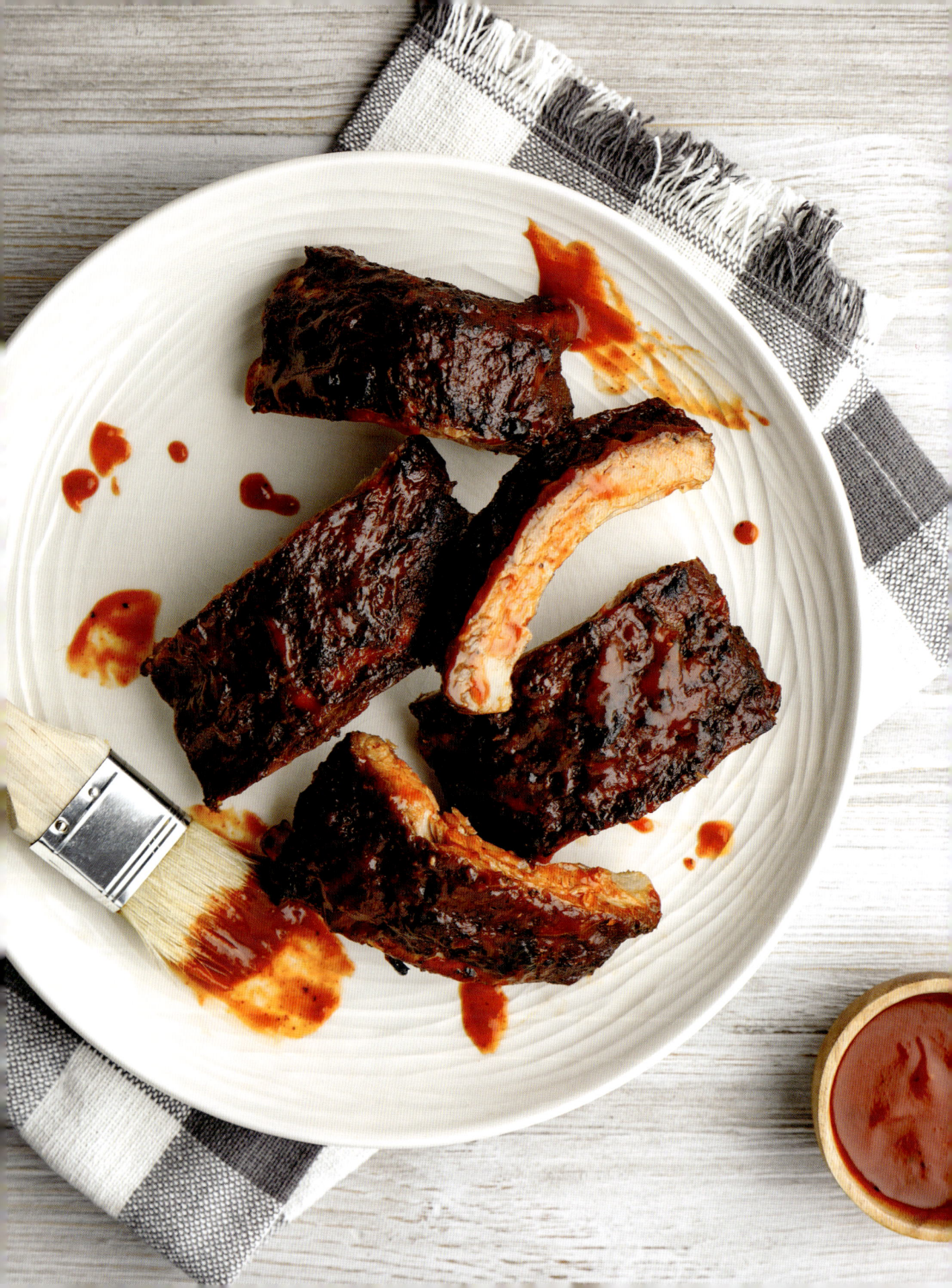

Prep Time: 15 min | High Pressure: 35 min | Natural Release: 15 min | Serves: 4

# Baby Back Ribs

Done in just under an hour, these ribs are falling off the bone and packed with all the flavor of a backyard barbeque, without having to spend an entire afternoon cooking.

## Ingredients

1 cup chicken stock
1 tablespoon cider vinegar
1 rack baby back ribs (about 2 pounds)
1 tablespoon smoked paprika
1 teaspoon salt
3/4 teaspoon pepper

### Barbecue Sauce

1 (8-ounce) can tomato sauce
2 tablespoons tomato paste
1/4 cup sugar substitute
1 tablespoon cider vinegar
1 1/2 teaspoons liquid smoke
1 1/2 teaspoons Worcestershire sauce
1/2 teaspoon onion powder
3/4 teaspoon salt
1/2 teaspoon pepper

### Special Equipment

Steam rack

1. Pour chicken stock and cider vinegar into the Instant Pot and place a steam rack over top.

2. For the easiest ribs to eat, flip rack over and locate a thin skin on the underside. Slip a butter knife under the skin to loosen it, then use your hands to pull it off the entire rack.

3. Season the entire surface of the ribs with smoked paprika, salt, and pepper.

4. Whisk together all Barbecue Sauce ingredients and brush 1/4 of the sauce over top the ribs.

5. Place the ribs on the steam rack in the cooker by coiling them around the circumference of the cooker.

6. Lock lid in place and seal pressure release vent. Set cooker to HIGH pressure for 35 minutes.

7. Let pressure release naturally for 15 minutes before opening vent to release any remaining pressure.

8. Carefully transfer ribs to a sheet pan and brush with the remaining Barbecue Sauce.

9. Place under broiler for 5 minutes, watching closely, just until sauce has browned. Cut ribs into sections and serve immediately.

### Instant Tips

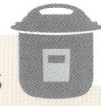

This recipe can actually be used to make 2 racks of ribs (coiling the second rack inside the first rack), but it will be a tight fit in a 6-quart cooker, so this is only recommended with smaller ribs.

---

Calories: 490 | Fat: 32g | Protein: 39.5g | Total Carbs: 8g - Fiber: 1.5g = Net Carbs: 6.5g

**Prep Time:** 10 min | **High Pressure:** 60 min | **Natural Release:** 15 min | **Serves:** 6

# Jamaican Jerk Pork Shoulder

While Jamaican Jerk traditionally requires the meat to be cooked slowly over a smoking wood fire, you can get very close to the same results here in just a fraction of the time, with all the island flavors you crave.

## Ingredients

- 2 tablespoons olive oil
- 1 (3 to 4-pound) pork shoulder roast
- 2 tablespoons jerk seasoning
- 1 cup chicken stock
- 1 tablespoon minced garlic
- 1 teaspoon lime zest
- 1 teaspoon sugar substitute

1. Heat olive oil in the Instant Pot on the SAUTÉ setting.
2. Generously season roast with jerk seasoning on all sides, rubbing it into the meat.
3. Add the seasoned roast to the cooker and brown well on at least 2 sides.
4. Whisk together chicken stock, garlic, lime zest, and sugar substitute before pouring over the roast in the cooker.
5. Lock lid in place and seal pressure release vent. Set cooker to HIGH pressure for 60 minutes.
6. Let pressure release naturally for 15 minutes before opening vent to release any remaining pressure.
7. Using two large forks, pull the meat into thick chunks and serve drizzled with the liquid from the cooker.

*Meats*

### Instant Tips

Make your own jerk seasoning by combining 1 tablespoon salt, 2 teaspoons dried thyme, 2 teaspoons onion powder, 2 teaspoons garlic powder, 1 teaspoon cayenne pepper, 1 teaspoon paprika, 1 teaspoon allspice, $\frac{1}{2}$ teaspoon black pepper, $\frac{1}{4}$ teaspoon cinnamon, and $\frac{1}{4}$ teaspoon nutmeg.

**Calories:** 540 | **Fat:** 40.5g | **Protein:** 40.5g | **Total Carbs:** 0.5g - **Fiber:** 0g = **Net Carbs:** 0.5g

**Prep Time:** 15 min | **High Pressure:** 60 min | **Natural Release:** 15 min | **Serves:** 6

# Barbacoa Beef

Typically made with "chipotle peppers in adobo sauce" (which includes added sugar), we make this spicy shredded beef with chipotle chili powder, tomato paste, and sugar substitute instead. Serve over cauliflower rice as part of a "burrito bowl" or in lettuce wraps topped with your favorite taco fixings.

## Ingredients

- 2 tablespoons olive oil
- 1 (2-pound) chuck roast
- 1 tablespoon chipotle chili powder
- 2 teaspoons ground cumin
- 2 teaspoons dried oregano
- 1 1/2 teaspoons salt
- 1 teaspoon pepper
- 1/2 teaspoon ground cloves
- 1/4 cup minced red onion
- 1 tablespoon minced garlic
- 1/2 cup beef stock
- 3 tablespoons tomato paste
- 2 tablespoons cider vinegar
- 1 tablespoon sugar substitute
- 1 bay leaf

1. Heat olive oil in the Instant Pot on the SAUTÉ setting.
2. Cut the chuck roast into 4 equal-sized pieces and season all pieces with chipotle chili powder, cumin, oregano, salt, pepper, and cloves.
3. Add the seasoned roast pieces to the cooker and brown well on at least 2 sides.
4. Add onion and garlic to the cooker, tossing with the meat before adding beef stock, tomato paste, cider vinegar, sugar substitute, and bay leaf. Toss until the tomato paste is mostly incorporated into the liquid.
5. Lock lid in place and seal pressure release vent. Set cooker to HIGH pressure for 60 minutes.
6. Let pressure release naturally for 15 minutes before opening vent to release any remaining pressure.
7. Using two large forks, shred the beef directly into the liquid in the cooker before serving.

### Instant Tips

We like to squeeze a splash of fresh lime juice into the cooker right before serving topped with diced red onion and chopped cilantro.

**Calories:** 440 | **Fat:** 33g | **Protein:** 29.5g | **Total Carbs:** 5g - **Fiber:** 1.5g = **Net Carbs:** 3.5g

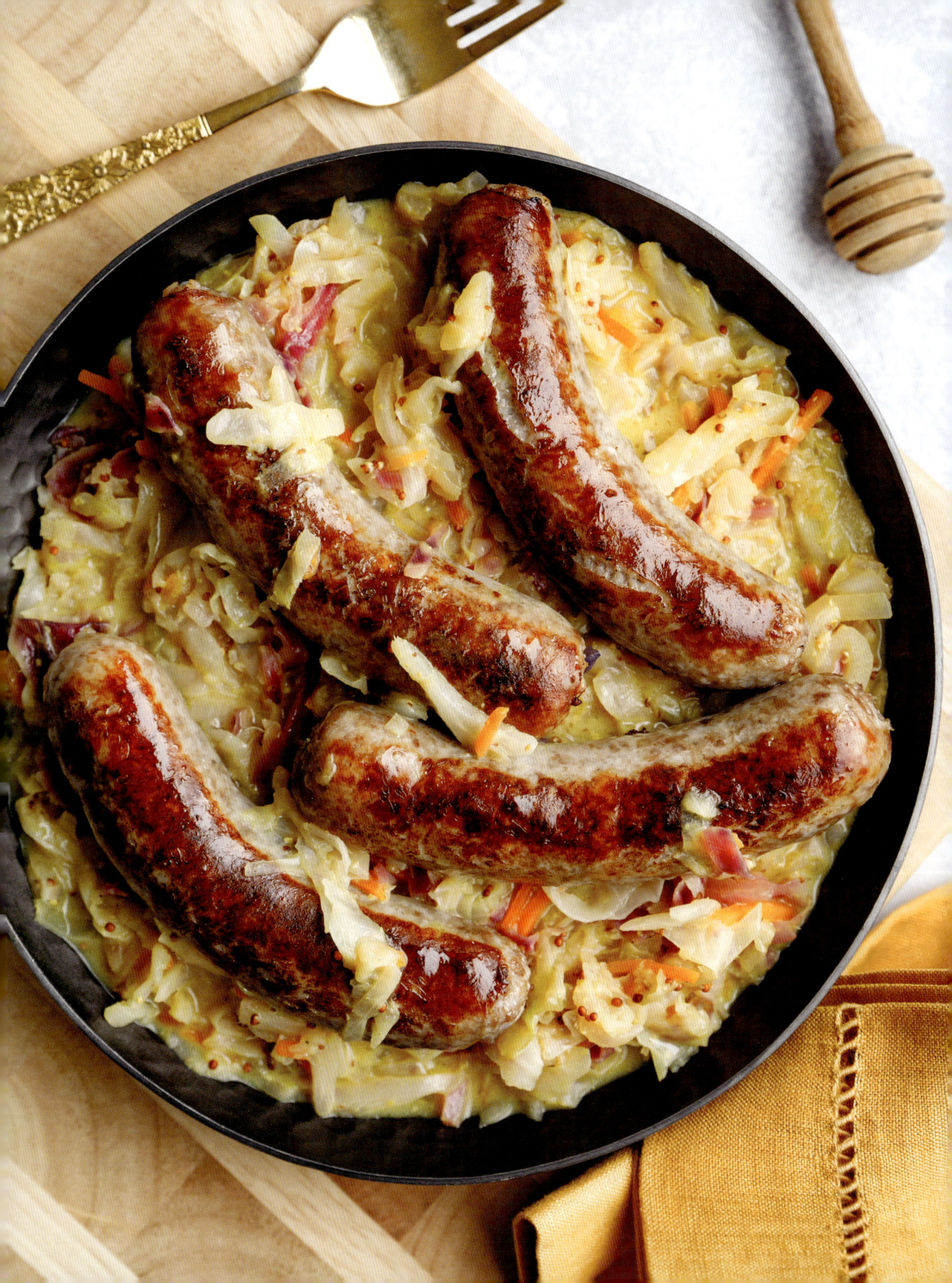

Prep Time: 10 min | High Pressure: 6 min | Quick Release | Serves: 5

# Bratwurst with Honey Mustard Kraut

The sweet and tangy mustard flavor in this kraut makes for a great alternative for those who aren't big fans of traditional sauerkraut but still want the perfect side for a perfectly cooked bratwurst.

## Ingredients

1 tablespoon vegetable oil

5 links fresh bratwurst

½ yellow onion, sliced

¾ cup chicken stock

2 tablespoons sugar substitute

1 tablespoon cider vinegar

16 ounces shredded coleslaw cabbage mix

3 tablespoons whole grain mustard

3 tablespoons yellow mustard

1 tablespoon butter

1. Heat vegetable oil in the Instant Pot on the SAUTÉ setting.

2. Place bratwurst in cooker and brown well on 2 sides. Remove from cooker and set aside.

3. Add onion to the cooker and cook just until translucent, about 2 minutes.

4. Add chicken stock, sugar substitute, and cider vinegar and stir to combine. Top with the shredded coleslaw cabbage, then place browned bratwurst over top of cabbage.

5. Lock lid in place and seal pressure release vent. Set cooker to HIGH pressure for 6 minutes.

6. Carefully open vent to quickly release the pressure.

7. Set aside bratwurst and stir whole grain mustard, yellow mustard, and butter into the kraut before serving.

### Instant Tips

While it is best with bratwurst, the Honey Mustard Kraut in this recipe also will go well with fresh Italian sausage, which can be prepared using the same directions.

Calories: 350 | Fat: 27g | Protein: 15g | Total Carbs: 9g - Fiber: 2g = Net Carbs: 7g

Prep Time: 15 min | High Pressure: 30 min | Natural Release: 10 min | Serves: 4–6

# Beef Paprikash

Our version of the beloved Hungarian dish features chunks of beef stewed with onion, fresh dill, and plenty of sweet paprika, giving the tomato-based broth its namesake and signature flavor.

## Ingredients

1 tablespoon vegetable oil

1 tablespoon butter

1 1/2 pounds beef stew meat

Salt and pepper

1/2 cup diced yellow onion

1 1/2 tablespoons sweet paprika (see tip)

1/2 cup beef stock

2 tablespoons chopped fresh dill, divided

2 tablespoons tomato paste, divided

1/2 cup sour cream

1. Heat vegetable oil and butter in the Instant Pot on the SAUTÉ setting.

2. Generously season stew meat with salt and pepper before adding to the cooker and browning on at least one side.

3. Add the yellow onion and paprika and sauté with beef for 2 minutes or until fragrant.

4. Add the beef stock, 1 tablespoon of the dill, and 1 tablespoon of the tomato paste and stir to combine.

5. Lock lid in place and seal pressure release vent. Set cooker to HIGH pressure for 30 minutes.

6. Let pressure release naturally for 10 minutes before opening vent to release any remaining pressure.

7. Drain 3/4 of the liquid from the cooker before stirring in sour cream, the remaining tablespoon of dill, and remaining tablespoon of tomato paste.

8. Season with salt and pepper to taste before serving.

### Instant Tips

Sweet paprika may also be labeled as "Hungarian paprika." It's more flavorful and sweeter (without added sugar) than ordinary paprika. That said, regular paprika, or even smoked paprika, can be used in this dish in a pinch.

Calories: 440 | Fat: 30.5g | Protein: 33.5g | Total Carbs: 4.5g - Fiber: 1g = Net Carbs: 3.5g

**Prep Time:** 15 min | **High Pressure:** 50 min | **Natural Release:** 15 min | **Serves:** 6

# Greek Lamb Roast

Lamb is classically combined with mint, but here we've also added other Greek flavors of oregano, garlic, and a bit of fresh lemon to brighten things up.

## Ingredients

2 tablespoons olive oil

1 (2 to 3-pound) boneless lamb shoulder, cut in half

1 teaspoon dried oregano

1 teaspoon salt

¾ teaspoon pepper

¼ cup minced red onion

1 ½ tablespoons minced garlic

1 cup chicken stock

2 tablespoons chopped fresh oregano

Zest of 1 lemon

Juice of ½ lemon

2 tablespoons chopped fresh mint

1. Heat olive oil in the Instant Pot on the SAUTÉ setting.
2. Generously season lamb roast with the dried oregano, salt, and pepper before adding to the cooker and browning well on at least 2 sides.
3. Add the onion and garlic to the cooker in the empty spaces around the roast and let cook for 1 minute.
4. Pour in chicken stock and add the fresh oregano and lemon zest.
5. Lock lid in place and seal pressure release vent. Set cooker to HIGH pressure for 50 minutes.
6. Let pressure release naturally for 15 minutes before opening vent to release any remaining pressure. Transfer meat to a serving platter.
7. For the best flavor, use a spoon to skim any grease off the top of the liquid in the cooker. Set cooker to SAUTÉ and bring up to a simmer, letting cook until slightly reduced.
8. Turn off cooker and stir in lemon juice before seasoning with salt and pepper to taste.
9. Using two large forks, pull the roast into thick chunks. Serve drizzled with the liquid from the cooker and topped with fresh mint.

### Instant Tips

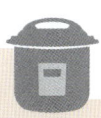

We also like to season the cooking liquid to taste with a tiny bit of sugar substitute to balance out the lemon and garlic.

---

**Calories:** 465 | **Fat:** 35g | **Protein:** 34g | **Total Carbs:** 1.5g - **Fiber:** 0.5g = **Net Carbs:** 1g

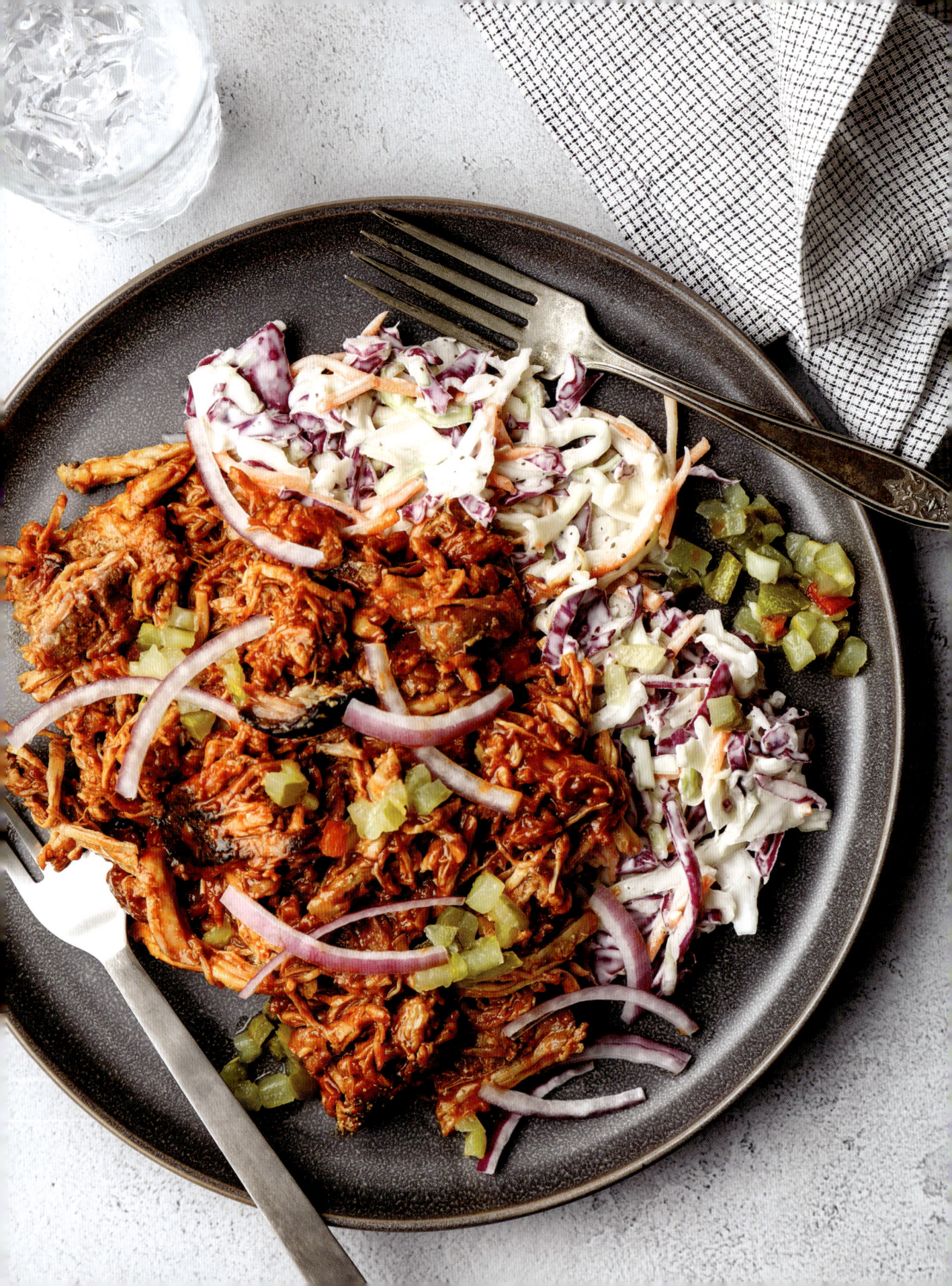

Prep Time: 15 min | High Pressure: 65 min | Natural Release: 15 min | Serves: 8

# Barbecue Pulled Pork

Pork roast is pulled into a homemade barbecue sauce that can turn any meal into a perfect indoor picnic. We like to serve this alongside fresh coleslaw, red onions, and dill pickles or dill pickle relish.

## Ingredients

2 tablespoons vegetable oil
1 (3 to 4-pound) pork shoulder roast
1 tablespoon smoked paprika
1 1/2 teaspoons salt
1 teaspoon pepper
1/2 teaspoon onion powder
1 cup chicken stock
1 tablespoon white vinegar

### Barbecue Sauce

1 (8-ounce) can tomato sauce
3 tablespoons sugar substitute
2 teaspoons white vinegar
1 1/2 teaspoons liquid smoke
1 teaspoon Worcestershire sauce
1 teaspoon minced garlic
1/2 teaspoon onion powder
3/4 teaspoon salt
1/2 teaspoon pepper

1. Heat vegetable oil in the Instant Pot on the SAUTÉ setting.
2. Cut the pork roast into 4 equal-sized pieces and season all pieces with smoked paprika, salt, pepper, and onion powder.
3. Add the seasoned roast pieces to the cooker and brown well on at least 2 sides. Pour in chicken stock and white vinegar.
4. Lock lid in place and seal pressure release vent. Set cooker to HIGH pressure for 65 minutes.
5. Let pressure release naturally for 15 minutes before opening vent to release any remaining pressure.
6. Meanwhile, whisk together all Barbecue Sauce ingredients to make the sauce.
7. Drain most of the liquid in the cooker and pour in Barbecue Sauce in its place.
8. Using two large forks, pull the meat into the sauce.
9. Set cooker to SAUTÉ and heat, stirring constantly, just until sauce is bubbly hot. Turn off cooker and serve immediately.

**Instant Tips**

You can also use a store-bought no-sugar-added barbecue sauce in place of the homemade version in this recipe.

Calories: 435 | Fat: 30g | Protein: 31g | Total Carbs: 8.5g - Fiber: 2g = Net Carbs: 6.5g

Instant Low Carb

Prep Time: 15 min | High Pressure: 75 min | Natural Release: 15 min | Serves: 8

# Sweet Onion Brisket

Caramelized onions and smoked paprika top this beef brisket for a sweet and smoky taste without barbecue sauce.

## Ingredients

1 tablespoon vegetable oil
1 tablespoon butter
1 small yellow onion, sliced
1 tablespoon smoked paprika
2 teaspoons chili powder
1/2 teaspoon pepper
1/4 teaspoon salt
1/2 cup beef stock
1/4 cup soy sauce
2 tablespoons sugar substitute
2 teaspoons Worcestershire sauce
1/2 teaspoon onion powder
1 (3 to 4-pound) beef brisket

1. Heat vegetable oil and butter in the Instant Pot on the SAUTÉ setting.

2. Add onion, smoked paprika, chili powder, pepper, and salt and sauté until the onion begins to brown. Remove from cooker and turn cooker off.

3. Add beef stock, soy sauce, sugar substitute, Worcestershire sauce, and onion powder to the empty cooker and stir to combine.

4. Place brisket into the liquid in the cooker, cutting it in half if necessary to fit.

5. Spread the seasoned and cooked onion evenly over top the brisket.

6. Lock lid in place and seal pressure release vent. Set cooker to HIGH pressure for 75 minutes.

7. Let pressure release naturally for 15 minutes before opening vent to release any remaining pressure.

8. Transfer brisket to a cutting board and cover with aluminum foil to rest for at least 10 minutes before slicing to serve, drizzled with liquid from the cooker.

*Meats*

**Instant Tips**
For more color and flavor, broil the cooked brisket until lightly browned before letting it rest.

Calories: 570 | Fat: 48g | Protein: 29.5g | Total Carbs: 1.5g - Fiber: 0g = Net Carbs: 1.5g

Prep Time: 15 min | High Pressure: 45 min | Natural Release: 15 min | Serves: 4

# Balsamic Braised Short Ribs

Beef short ribs are cooked to tender perfection with fresh thyme and the signature sweetness of balsamic vinegar. It's an entrée worthy of any fine restaurant, made right in your Instant Pot.

## Ingredients

2 tablespoons olive oil
4 chuck short ribs (about 2 pounds)
Salt and pepper
¼ cup diced shallot
2 teaspoons minced garlic
½ cup beef stock
3 tablespoons balsamic vinegar
2 tablespoons sugar substitute
4 sprigs fresh thyme
1 tablespoon butter

1. Heat olive oil in the Instant Pot on the SAUTÉ setting.
2. Generously season short ribs with salt and pepper on both sides and add to the cooker. Brown well on at least 1 side.
3. Add the shallot and garlic in any gaps around the meat and let cook for 1 minute.
4. Whisk together beef stock, balsamic vinegar, and sugar substitute and pour into the cooker.
5. Top each short rib with a sprig of thyme.
6. Lock lid in place and seal pressure release vent. Set cooker to HIGH pressure for 45 minutes.
7. Let pressure release naturally for 15 minutes before opening vent to release any remaining pressure. Transfer short ribs to a plate and cover with aluminum foil.
8. For the best flavor, use a spoon to skim grease off the top of the cooking liquid.
9. Set cooker to SAUTÉ and let cooking liquid simmer for 5 minutes. Turn cooker off and stir in butter before serving short ribs drizzled with the cooking liquid.

### Instant Tips

We like to add a small splash of additional balsamic vinegar as we are adding the butter, as most of the original balsamic has lost its acidity by this point.

Calories: 445 | Fat: 28g | Protein: 43.5g | Total Carbs: 3g - Fiber: 0g = Net Carbs: 3g

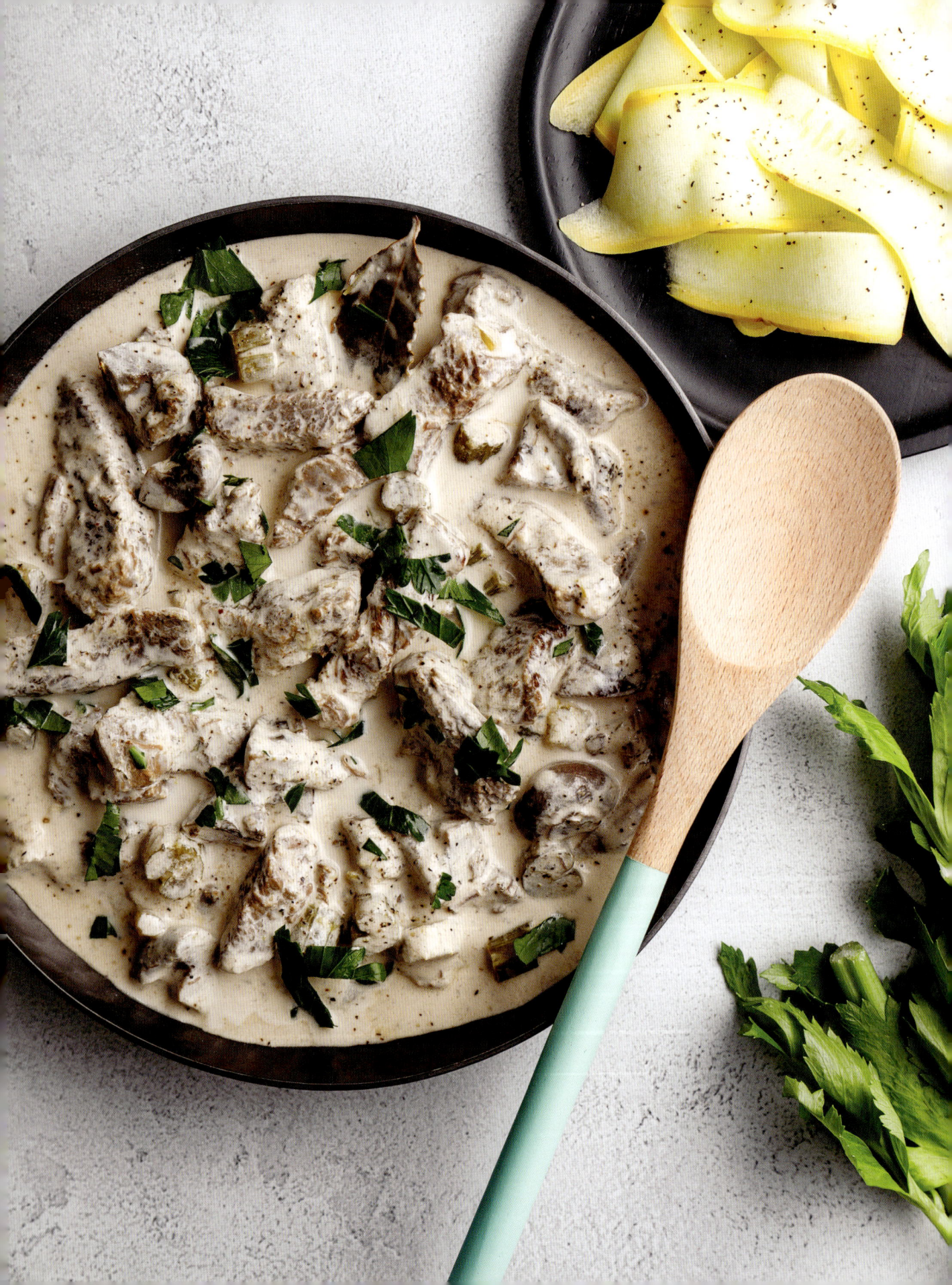

Prep Time: 15 min | High Pressure: 15 min | Natural Release: 5 min | Serves: 4

# Beef Stroganoff

In this recipe, tender strips of beef and baby bella mushrooms are simmered in the classic sour cream sauce you'd expect from a stroganoff. We like to serve this over ribbons of yellow squash in place of egg noodles.

## Ingredients

2 tablespoons vegetable oil

1 1/2 pounds top sirloin steak, cut into 3/4-inch thick strips

Salt and pepper

8 ounces baby bella mushrooms, quartered

3 stalks celery, chopped

1/2 cup diced red onion

2 teaspoons minced garlic

1 cup beef stock

1/4 cup sherry cooking wine

2 tablespoons Dijon mustard, divided

1 bay leaf

1/2 teaspoon dried thyme

1 cup sour cream

1/2 teaspoon celery salt

1/2 teaspoon pepper

Chopped parsley, for garnish

1. Heat vegetable oil in the Instant Pot on the SAUTÉ setting.

2. Generously season steak with salt and pepper before adding to the cooker and browning on at least one side.

3. Add the mushrooms, celery, onion, and garlic and sauté with steak for 2 minutes or until fragrant.

4. Add the beef stock, wine, 1 tablespoon of the mustard, bay leaf, and thyme and stir to combine.

5. Lock lid in place and seal pressure release vent. Set cooker to HIGH pressure for 15 minutes.

6. Let pressure release naturally for 5 minutes before opening vent to release any remaining pressure.

7. Drain 3/4 of the liquid from the cooker before stirring in sour cream, celery salt, pepper, and remaining tablespoon of mustard. Serve garnished with plenty of chopped parsley.

### Instant Tips

This is perfect when served over yellow squash or zucchini ribbons. To make these ribbons, simply shave the squash using a standard vegetable peeler! To cook, simply drop in boiling water for just 1 minute.

---

Calories: 460 | Fat: 28.5g | Protein: 38.5g | Total Carbs: 8.5g - Fiber: 1.5g = Net Carbs: 7g

Instant Low Carb • 129

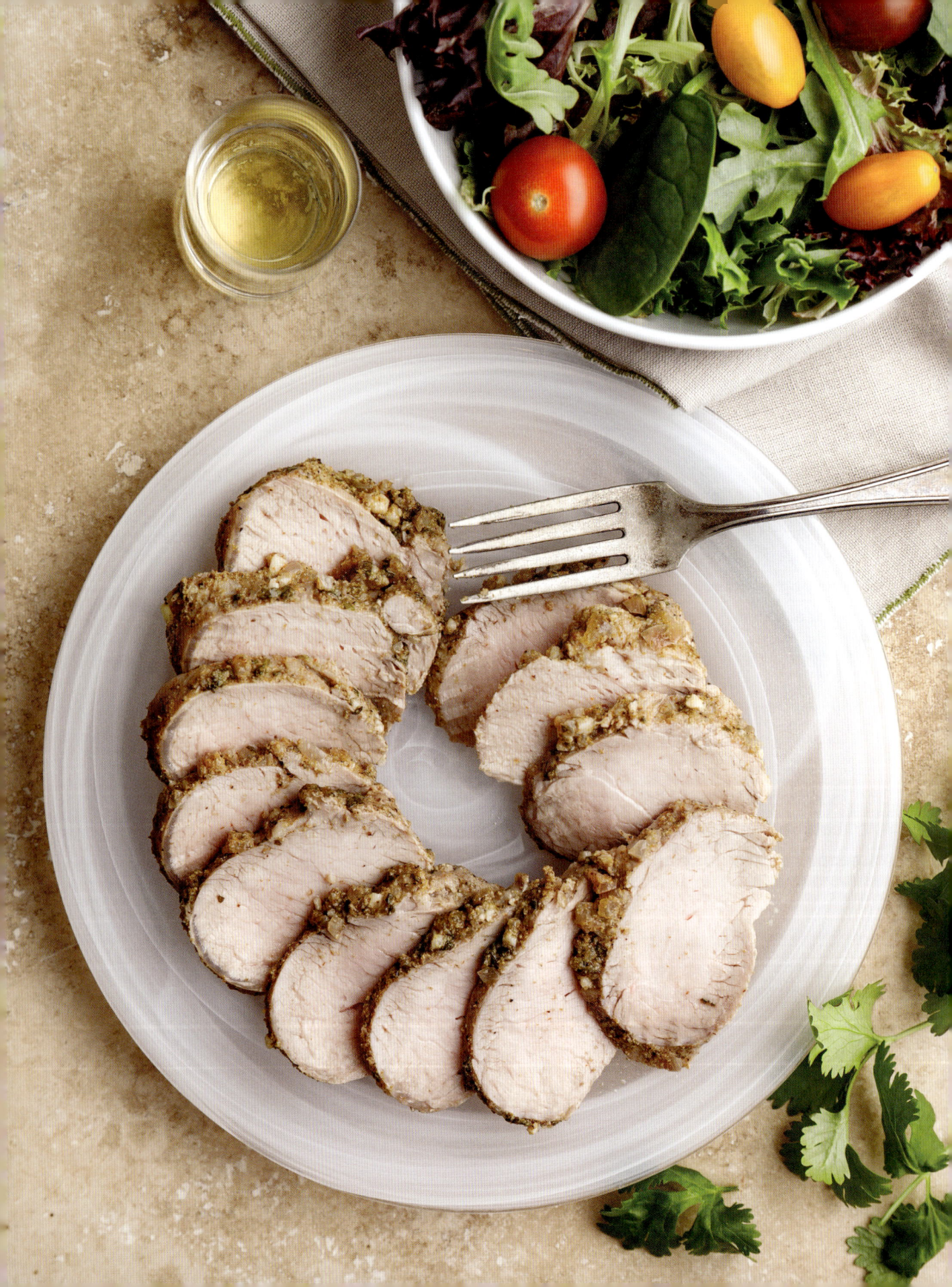

Prep Time: 10 min | High Pressure: 2 min | Natural Release: 10 min | Serves: 6

# Tequila Pork Tenderloin

Tequila Chicken has been one of our all-time most popular recipes for over a decade. Here, we've used the same flavorful cilantro and cumin rub on pork tenderloins, which cook to a perfect medium temperature in only 2 minutes (with a 10-minute natural release).

## Ingredients

1 cup chicken stock
3 tablespoons minced red onion
3 tablespoons chopped fresh cilantro
2 tablespoons tequila
1 1/2 tablespoons ground cumin
1 tablespoon extra-virgin olive oil
2 teaspoons minced garlic
1 teaspoon salt
3/4 teaspoon pepper
1/4 teaspoon onion powder
1/8 teaspoon cayenne pepper
2 pork tenderloins

## Special Equipment

Steam rack

1. Pour chicken stock into Instant Pot and place a steam rack over top.
2. In a small bowl, combine the red onion, cilantro, tequila, cumin, olive oil, garlic, salt, pepper, onion powder, and cayenne pepper.
3. Rub the spice mixture into all sides of each pork tenderloin before placing on the steam rack in the cooker.
4. Lock lid in place and seal pressure release vent. Set cooker to HIGH pressure for 2 minutes.
5. Let pressure release naturally for 10 minutes before opening vent to release any remaining pressure.
6. Use a meat thermometer to check for doneness. As long as it reads 145° F or above, the pork is done. If pork is under 145° F, secure the cooker's lid without turning it on and let the residual heat continue cooking the pork for 2 minutes at a time, just until it reaches temperature.
7. Let pork rest 10 minutes before slicing to serve.

### Instant Tips

Be sure to purchase fresh pork tenderloins that are not marinated or flavored. Fresh tenderloins almost always come in a pack of two.

Calories: 340 | Fat: 8g | Protein: 56.5g | Total Carbs: 1.5g - Fiber: 0g = Net Carbs: 1.5g

Prep Time: 15 min | High Pressure: 6 min | Quick Release | Serves: 5

# Italian Sausage with Peppers and Kale

As flavorful one-pot meals are always appreciated, these Italian sausages with super nutritious—and delicious—kale, red and green bell peppers, and red onion should become a colorful lunchtime staple!

## Ingredients

- 1 tablespoon olive oil
- 5 links fresh Italian sausage
- 1/2 red onion, sliced
- 1/2 green bell pepper, sliced
- 1/2 red bell pepper, sliced
- 1 tablespoon minced garlic
- 1/2 cup chicken stock
- 2 teaspoons lemon juice
- 1/4 teaspoon salt
- 1/4 teaspoon crushed red pepper flakes
- 4 packed cups chopped kale
- 1/4 cup grated Parmesan cheese

1. Heat olive oil in the Instant Pot on the SAUTÉ setting.
2. Place sausage in cooker and brown well on 2 sides. Remove from cooker and set aside.
3. Add onion, bell peppers, and garlic to the cooker and sauté just until vegetables begin to sweat, about 2 minutes.
4. Add chicken stock, lemon juice, salt, and red pepper flakes and stir to combine. Top with the kale, then place browned sausage over top kale.
5. Lock lid in place and seal pressure release vent. Set cooker to HIGH pressure for 6 minutes.
6. Carefully open vent to quickly release the pressure.
7. Serve sausage smothered in the kale, onion, and peppers, topped with grated Parmesan cheese.

### Instant Tips

We like hot Italian sausage in this. If using "sweet" sausage, check for added sugar in the ingredients.

Calories: 330 | Fat: 24g | Protein: 20g | Total Carbs: 8.5g - Fiber: 1.5g = Net Carbs: 7g

**Prep Time:** 10 min | **High Pressure:** 75 min | **Natural Release:** 15 min | **Serves:** 6

# Red Wine Braised Beef

This chuck pot roast is cooked up in dry red wine with whole sprigs of fresh rosemary. It's a simple and more elevated take on your traditional pot roast.

## Ingredients

2 tablespoons olive oil

3 tablespoons butter, divided

1 (2.5 to 3.5-pound) chuck roast

Salt and pepper

1 cup chopped celery

½ cup chopped red onion

1 tablespoon minced garlic

1 cup dry red wine

2 teaspoons Worcestershire sauce

2 sprigs fresh rosemary

1 bay leaf

1 teaspoon sugar substitute

½ teaspoon Italian seasoning

1. Heat olive oil and 1 tablespoon of the butter in the Instant Pot on the SAUTÉ setting.

2. Generously season roast with salt and pepper on both sides. For larger roasts that are over 3 pounds, cut in half for the most tender results.

3. Add the seasoned roast to the cooker and brown well on both sides. Remove from pot and set aside.

4. Add the celery, onion, and garlic to the cooker and sauté for 2 minutes or until vegetables begin to sweat.

5. Stir red wine, Worcestershire sauce, rosemary, bay leaf, sugar substitute, and Italian seasoning into the cooker.

6. Return browned roast to the cooker. Lock lid in place and seal pressure release vent. Set cooker to HIGH pressure for 75 minutes.

7. Let pressure release naturally for 15 minutes before opening vent to release any remaining pressure. Transfer roast to a plate and cover with aluminum foil.

8. Set cooker to SAUTÉ and let simmer 10 minutes or until braising liquid in the cooker has reduced by about ⅓.

9. Turn off cooker, stir in remaining 2 tablespoons of butter, and generously season braising liquid with salt and pepper to taste. Return roast to the cooker before pulling apart to serve drizzled with braising liquid.

**Instant Tips**

This is also delicious with ¼ cup of heavy cream added to the braising liquid in the last step.

**Calories:** 540 | **Fat:** 40g | **Protein:** 36.5g | **Total Carbs:** 2.5g - **Fiber:** 0.5g = **Net Carbs:** 2g

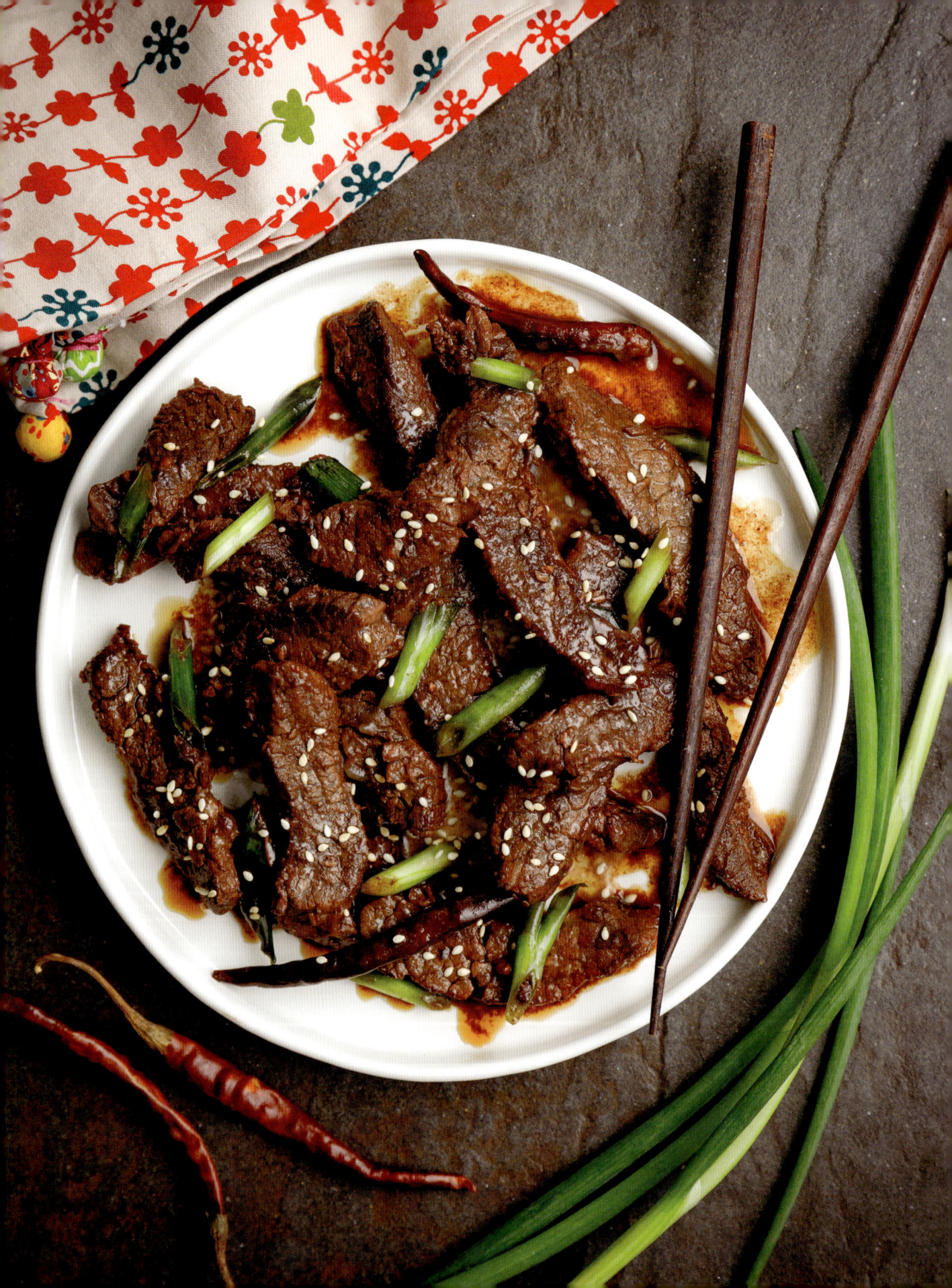

**Prep Time: 15 min | High Pressure: 20 min | Natural Release: 10 min | Serves: 4**

# Mongolian Beef

Sliced flank steak is tossed with scallions, fresh ginger, and a hint of dried chili peppers in a sweet, savory, and spicy sauce that's just like takeout—without the carbs.

## Ingredients

- 2 tablespoons sesame oil, divided
- 1 1/2 pounds flank steak, sliced into 1/2-inch thick strips
- 2 teaspoons Chinese five-spice powder
- 1 tablespoon minced garlic
- 1 tablespoon minced fresh ginger
- 1/3 cup beef stock
- 2 tablespoons soy sauce
- 3 tablespoons sugar substitute
- 1 tablespoon rice wine vinegar
- 3 dried red chili peppers
- 4 scallions, chopped

1. Heat 1 tablespoon of the sesame oil in the Instant Pot on the SAUTÉ setting.
2. Add steak to the cooker and toss in five-spice powder. Cook until browned on at least one side.
3. Add the garlic and ginger and sauté with steak for 2 minutes or until fragrant.
4. Stir in beef stock, soy sauce, sugar substitute, rice wine vinegar, and dried chili peppers.
5. Lock lid in place and seal pressure release vent. Set cooker to HIGH pressure for 20 minutes.
6. Let pressure release naturally for 10 minutes before opening vent to release any remaining pressure.
7. Set cooker to SAUTÉ and bring up to a simmer. Let simmer until the liquid has reduced by 1/3 and is beginning to coat the meat.
8. Stir in scallions and the remaining tablespoon of sesame oil before serving.

### Instant Tips

To make this into a meal, add a bag of frozen broccoli florets after pressure cooking as you are reducing the sauce.

---

**Calories: 360 | Fat: 22g | Protein: 37.5g | Total Carbs: 4.5g - Fiber: 0.5g = Net Carbs: 4g**

Prep Time: 10 min | High Pressure: 25 min | Natural Release: 15 min | Serves: 4

# Boneless Ribs with Sweet Chili Sauce

These boneless country-style ribs have a sauce that is a cross between Chinese sweet-and-sour sauce and chili garlic sauce with crushed red pepper. Be warned, it can be a bit spicy!

## Ingredients

1 cup chicken stock

2 pounds boneless country-style pork ribs

### Sweet Chili Sauce

3 tablespoons tomato paste

2 tablespoons soy sauce

2 tablespoons sugar substitute

2 tablespoons cider vinegar

1 tablespoon sesame oil

2 teaspoons minced garlic

1 teaspoon crushed red pepper flakes

### Special Equipment

Steam rack

1. Pour chicken stock into the Instant Pot and place a steam rack over top.
2. In a large mixing bowl, whisk together all Sweet Chili Sauce ingredients. Remove $1/2$ of the sauce and set aside for after you cook the ribs (to prevent cross-contamination).
3. Add ribs to the large mixing bowl and toss in the first $1/2$ of the sauce before placing the coated ribs on the steam rack in the cooker.
4. Lock lid in place and seal pressure release vent. Set cooker to HIGH pressure for 25 minutes.
5. Let pressure release naturally for 15 minutes before opening vent to release any remaining pressure.
6. Carefully transfer ribs to a sheet pan and brush with the remaining $1/2$ of the Sweet Chili Sauce.
7. Place under broiler, watching closely, just until sauce has browned.

**Meats**

### Instant Tips

If you aren't a fan of spicy food, you will definitely want to lower the crushed red pepper flakes in this sauce down to only a small pinch.

Calories: 310 | Fat: 11.5g | Protein: 49g | Total Carbs: 2.5g - Fiber: 0.5g = Net Carbs: 2g

**Prep Time: 15 min** | **High Pressure: 65 min** | **Natural Release: 15 min** | **Serves: 8**

# Pork Carnitas

This Mexican pulled pork is unique in that the end result is both tender and crispy. To make it a meal, try serving these carnitas in lettuce wraps, sprinkled with chopped cilantro. Make sure to have plenty of fresh lime wedges to squeeze over top.

## Ingredients

- 2 tablespoons olive oil
- 1 (3 to 4-pound) pork shoulder roast
- 1 tablespoon chipotle chili powder
- 2 teaspoons ground cumin
- 1 ½ teaspoons salt
- 1 teaspoon pepper
- 1 teaspoon dried oregano
- ⅓ cup minced yellow onion
- 1 tablespoon minced garlic
- ½ cup chicken stock
- 1 (4-ounce) can diced green chiles
- Zest of ½ lime
- Juice of 1 lime
- 1 bay leaf

1. Heat olive oil in the Instant Pot on the SAUTÉ setting.
2. Cut the pork roast into 4 equal-sized pieces and season all pieces with chipotle chili powder, cumin, salt, pepper, and oregano.
3. Add the seasoned roast pieces to the cooker and brown well on at least 2 sides.
4. Add onion and garlic to the cooker, tossing with the meat before adding chicken stock, green chiles, lime zest, lime juice, and bay leaf.
5. Lock lid in place and seal pressure release vent. Set cooker to HIGH pressure for 65 minutes.
6. Let pressure release naturally for 15 minutes before opening vent to release any remaining pressure.
7. Transfer pork to a sheet pan and use two forks to pull the meat into small shreds.
8. Place sheet pan under broiler for 5 minutes or until meat begins to crisp.
9. Drizzle the pulled and crisped meat with plenty of liquid from the cooker before serving.

### Instant Tips

Traditional carnitas are nice and crispy. You can better replicate this texture by removing the crisped meat from the broiler, tossing in liquid from the cooker, then broiling a second time.

**Calories: 410** | **Fat: 30.5g** | **Protein: 30g** | **Total Carbs: 2g** - **Fiber: 0.5g** = **Net Carbs: 1.5g**

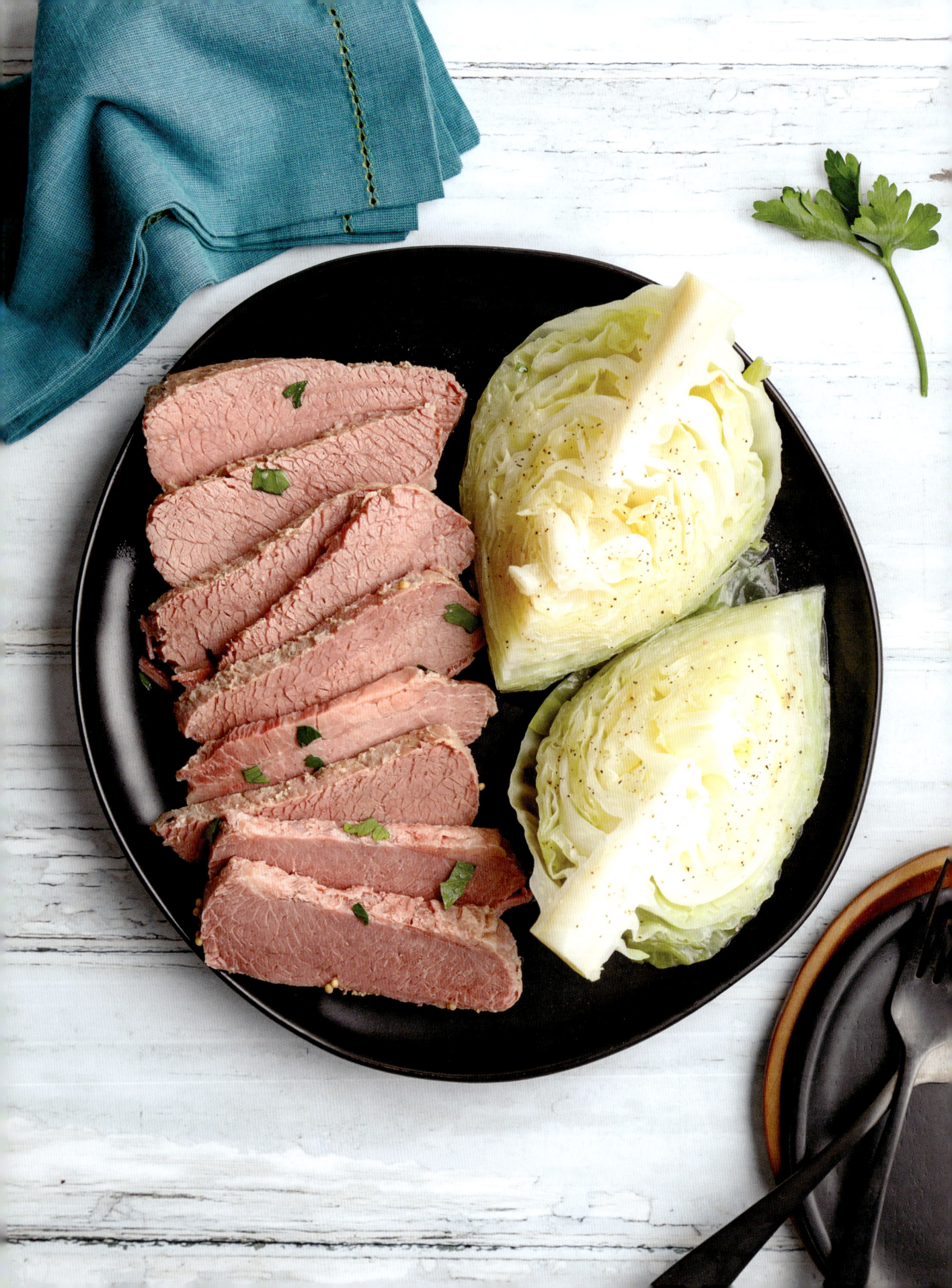

Prep Time: 5 min | High Pressure: 75 min | Natural Release: 15 min | Serves: 8

# Corned Beef and Cabbage

Now you can enjoy an Irish dinner in far, far less time than oven or stovetop preparations. We've found that 75 minutes under pressure with a 15 minute natural release makes for corned beef that is tender but not so tender that the meat falls apart as you slice it.

## Ingredients

1 (3 to 4-pound) corned beef with pickling spice packet

2 teaspoons minced garlic

2 teaspoons vegetable oil

12 ounces low-carb beer, optional

1 head cabbage, cut into 8 wedges

1. Place corned beef in Instant Pot and empty pickling spice packet over top. Add garlic and vegetable oil.
2. Pour beer into cooker, if desired, before filling cooker with enough water to cover the entire corned beef without exceeding the max-fill line.
3. Lock lid in place and seal pressure release vent. Set cooker to HIGH pressure for 75 minutes.
4. Let pressure release naturally for 15 minutes before opening vent to release any remaining pressure.
5. Transfer corned beef to a cutting board and cover with aluminum foil to rest for at least 10 minutes.
6. Meanwhile, add cabbage to the liquid in the Instant Pot.
7. Lock lid in place and seal pressure release vent. Set cooker to HIGH pressure for 3 minutes.
8. Carefully open vent to quickly release the pressure. Carve the rested meat and serve alongside cabbage, drizzled with liquid from the cooker.

**Instant Tips**

If the meat has overly cooled or begins to dry out as you carve it, simply dip into the hot liquid in the cooker before serving.

Calories: 390 | Fat: 29g | Protein: 26g | Total Carbs: 5.5g - Fiber: 2g = Net Carbs: 3.5g

*Chapter 6*

# Seafood & Sauté

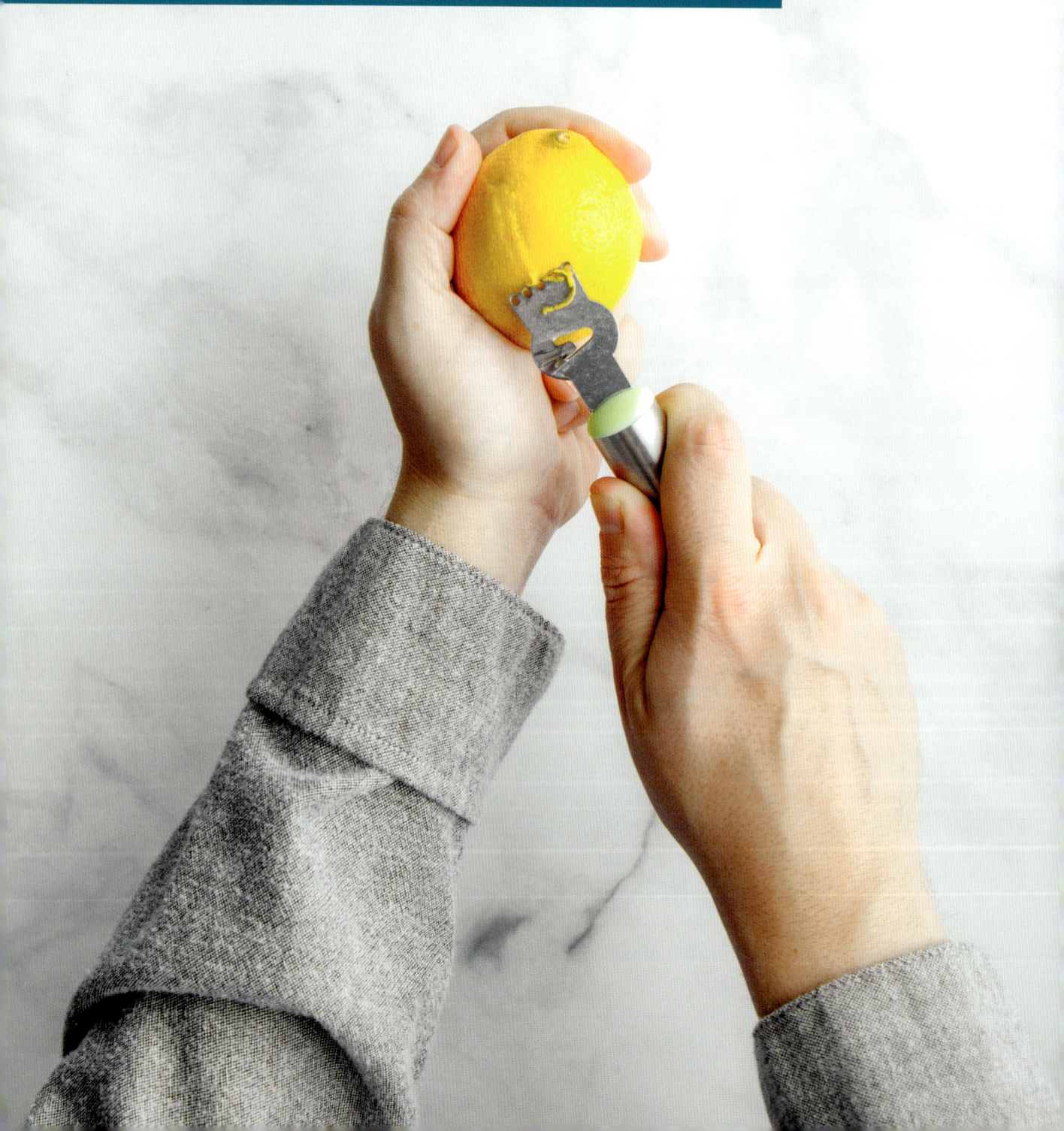

## recipes in this chapter...

**Simple Salmon Fillets with Dill, 143**

**Chicken and Shrimp Gumbo, 144**

**Zucchini in Clam Sauce, 145**

**Cauliflower Risotto with Shrimp, 147**

**Scallops with Capers and Dill, 149**

**Spinach with Artichokes, 150**

**Ground Turkey Bolognese, 151**

**Instant Popcorn, 153**

**Cauliflower Fried Rice with Ham, 154**

**Margherita Chicken with Spaghetti Squash, 155**

**Indian-Spiced Cashews, 157**

**Snap Peas with Crispy Pancetta, 158**

**Cheesy Ground Beef Skillet, 159**

**Red Bliss Radishes, 161**

Secret Message #6: The lemon photo on the opposite page was shot at 11:57 p.m. on New Year's Eve. We took it and then watched Disney World's fireworks from our backyard.

Sauté

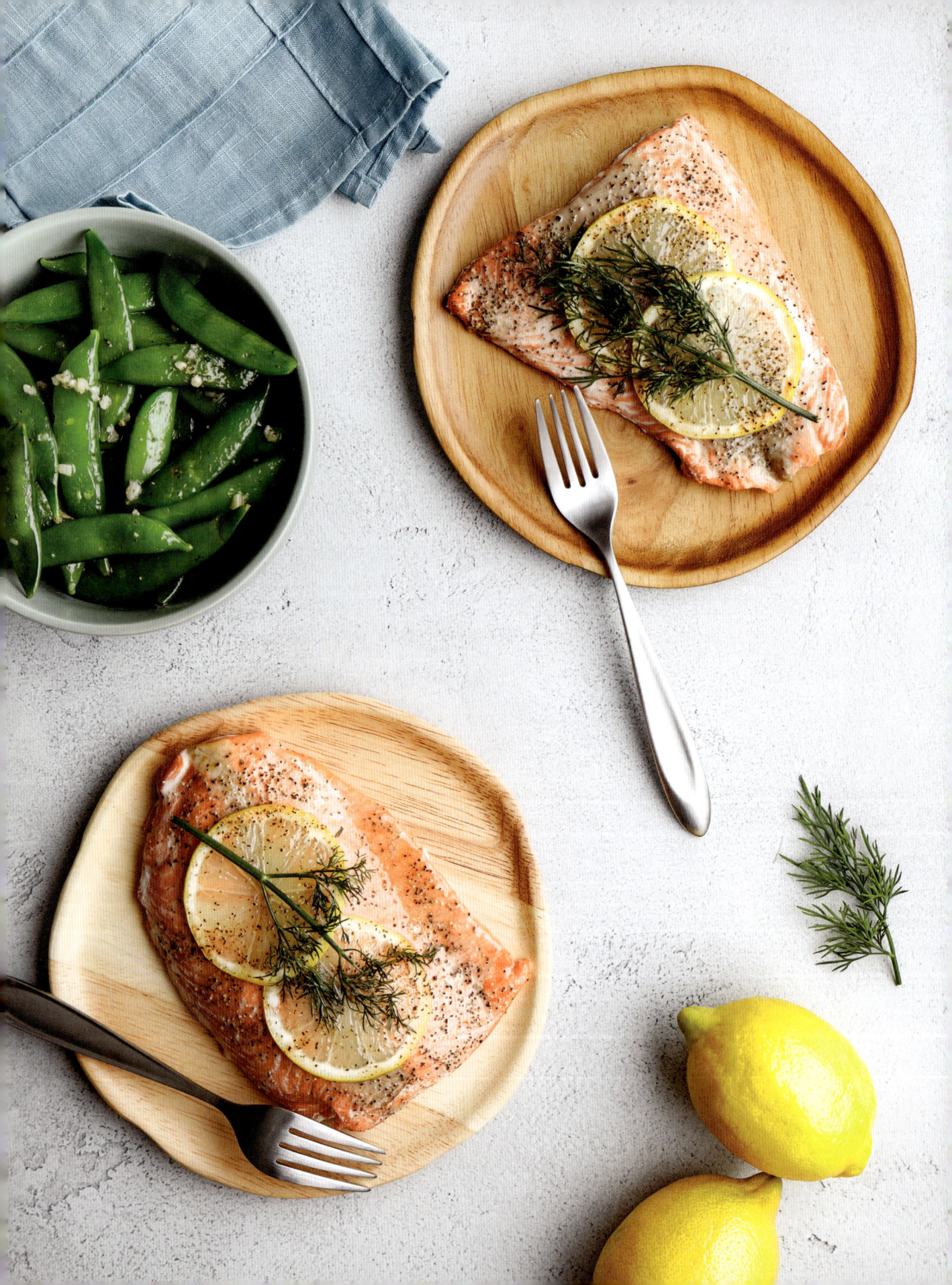

Prep Time: 5 min | High Pressure: 5 min | Quick Release | Serves: 2

# Simple Salmon Fillets with Dill

When it comes to cooking under pressure, we've learned that using frozen fillets of salmon is far safer than using fresh, as fresh salmon can easily overcook depending on the thickness. With frozen salmon, we ensure a perfect fillet each and every time.

## Ingredients

Juice of ½ lemon
1 sprig fresh dill, optional
2 frozen salmon fillets
Salt and pepper
1 tablespoon chopped fresh dill
2 slices lemon
Melted butter, optional

## Special Equipment

Steam rack

1. Pour 1 cup of water into the Instant Pot, add the juice of ½ lemon, and insert a steam rack over top. For more flavor, add a sprig of dill to the water.

2. Place the salmon fillets on the steam rack and season generously with salt and pepper.

3. Sprinkle with the chopped dill, then top each fillet with a slice of lemon.

4. Lock lid in place and seal pressure release vent. Set cooker to HIGH pressure for 5 minutes.

5. Carefully open vent to quickly release the pressure.

6. Serve immediately. For more flavor, drizzle with a bit of melted butter before serving.

*Sauté*

### Instant Tips

You can cook up to 3 salmon fillets this way, but 4 will be a tight fit. You are looking for the type of frozen salmon that comes in a bag with individually wrapped fillets inside, not anything in a box that may already be seasoned.

Calories: 385 | Fat: 27g | Protein: 34g | Total Carbs: 0.5g - Fiber: 0g = Net Carbs: 0.5g

Prep Time: 20 min | High Pressure: 2 min | Quick Release | Serves: 6

# Chicken and Shrimp Gumbo

The zesty flavors of this Creole stew are a taste of New Orleans. A trio of chicken, shrimp, and andouille sausage is combined with the classic vegetable trinity of bell pepper, celery, and onion in a tomato-based sauce. Cauliflower rice is then mixed right in, making this a complete meal.

## Ingredients

3 tablespoons butter

1 tablespoon vegetable oil

1 pound boneless, skinless chicken breasts, chopped

8 ounces smoked andouille sausage, chopped

1 green bell pepper, chopped

½ cup chopped yellow onion

3 stalks celery, chopped

1 tablespoon minced garlic

1 tablespoon Creole seasoning

1 (14.5-ounce) can petite diced tomatoes, with liquid

2 cups chicken broth

2 bay leaves

¼ teaspoon crushed red pepper flakes

1 pound peeled and deveined shrimp

2 cups grated cauliflower (cauliflower rice)

Chopped parsley, to top

1. Heat butter and vegetable oil in the Instant Pot on the SAUTÉ setting.
2. Add chicken, sausage, bell pepper, onion, celery, garlic, and Creole seasoning to the cooker and sauté 5 minutes.
3. Stir in diced tomatoes, chicken broth, bay leaves, and red pepper flakes.
4. Lock lid in place and seal pressure release vent. Set cooker to HIGH pressure for 2 minutes.
5. Carefully open vent to quickly release the pressure.
6. Set Instant Pot to SAUTÉ, add shrimp and cauliflower, and bring up to a simmer. Let simmer 5 minutes or until shrimp are opaque throughout and cauliflower is tender.
7. Season with additional Creole seasoning to taste before serving topped with plenty of chopped parsley.

*Sauté*

**Instant Tips**

Most stores carry andouille sausage, but in a pinch, any type of smoked sausage can be used in its place.

Calories: 385 | Fat: 21.5g | Protein: 39g | Total Carbs: 8.5g - Fiber: 2g = Net Carbs: 6.5g

Prep Time: 20 min | Cook Time: 5 min | Sauté | Serves: 4

# Zucchini in Clam Sauce

The clam sauce for these zucchini "zoodles" is made in mere minutes thanks to canned baby clams (both whole and minced). While canned clams may not seem fancy, they're the same thing they are using to make Linguine in Clam Sauce at most Mom and Pop Italian restaurants. It's extremely expensive and labor intensive to make it using fresh clams. Some canned seafood gets a bad rap, even though it really isn't any different than putting tuna in a can!

## Ingredients

3 tablespoons butter
2 tablespoons olive oil
3 tablespoons minced red onion
1 1/2 tablespoons minced garlic
1/3 cup dry white wine
1/2 teaspoon pepper
1/4 teaspoon salt
1/4 teaspoon crushed red pepper flakes
1 (10-ounce) can whole baby clams, drained
1 (6.5-ounce) can minced baby clams, drained
4 zucchini, spiralized
Chopped fresh parsley, to top

1. Heat butter and olive oil in the Instant Pot on the SAUTÉ setting.
2. Add red onion and garlic and sauté 2 minutes or until the garlic begins to slightly darken in color.
3. Stir in white wine, pepper, salt, and red pepper flakes and bring up to a simmer. Let simmer 1 minute.
4. Stir in clams and zucchini and let cook 1 additional minute. Turn off heat, cover, and let rest 1 minute or until zucchini is tender.
5. Serve topped with plenty of fresh parsley.

### Instant Tips

For a richer sauce, add a splash of heavy cream after adding the wine, but be sure to stir the sauce as it simmers.

Calories: 255 | Fat: 17g | Protein: 15.5g | Total Carbs: 8g - Fiber: 1.5g = Net Carbs: 6.5g

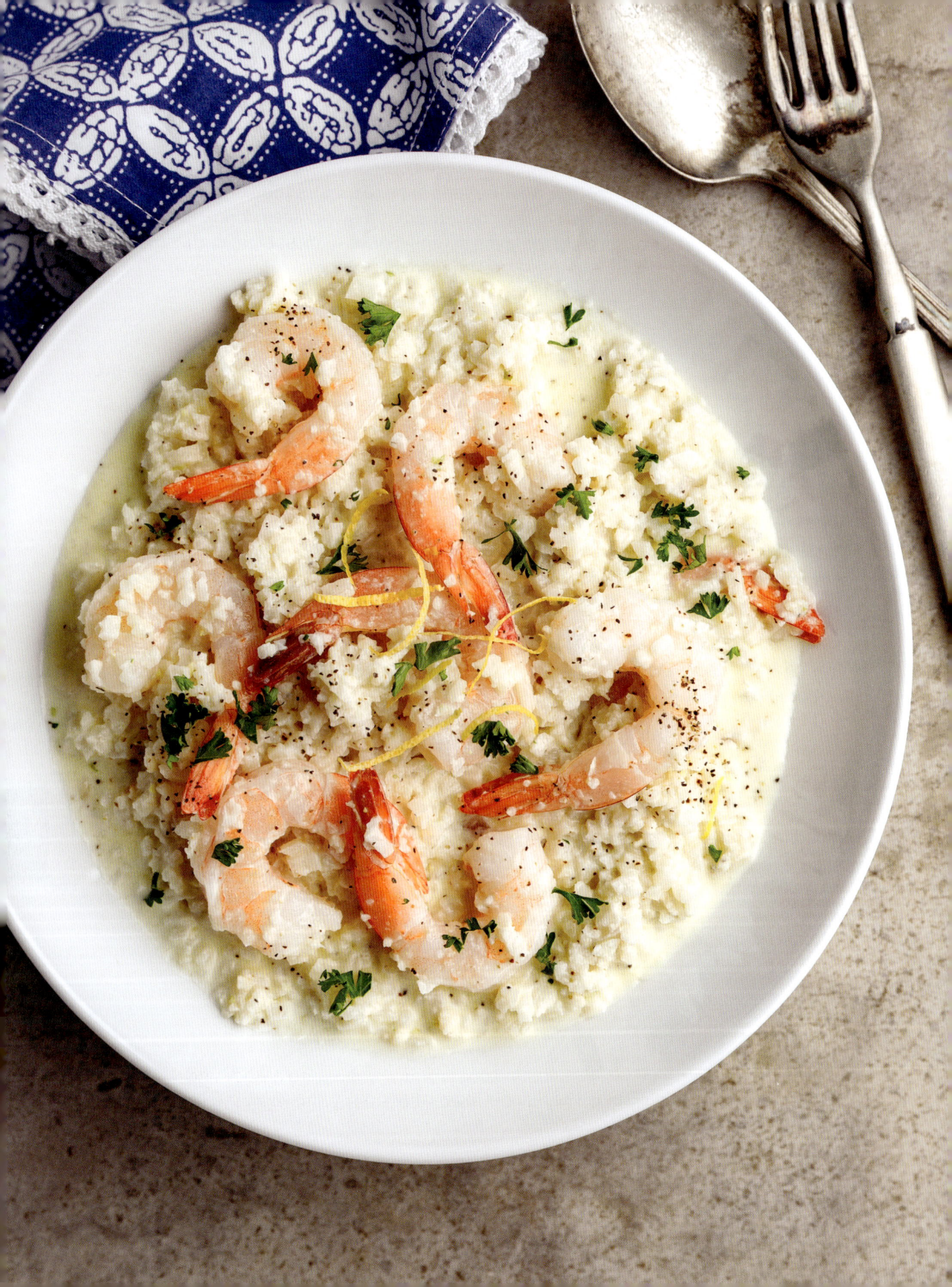

**Prep Time: 15 min | Cook Time: 12 min | Sauté | Serves: 4**

# Cauliflower Risotto with Shrimp

This recreation of risotto has shrimp and cauliflower in a creamy white wine sauce with Parmesan cheese. For the best texture, we finely grate fresh cauliflower florets in a food processor, as store-bought cauliflower rice (which will certainly work to save time) has bigger grains than what you'd find in a risotto.

## Ingredients

- 2 tablespoons vegetable oil
- 2 tablespoons butter
- 1 pound peeled and deveined shrimp
- 2 tablespoons minced red onion
- 1 tablespoon minced garlic
- 12–16 ounces grated cauliflower (cauliflower rice)
- ½ cup dry white wine
- ½ cup heavy cream
- ¼ cup grated Parmesan cheese
- ½ teaspoon salt
- ½ teaspoon pepper
- Chopped parsley, to top

1. Heat vegetable oil and butter in the Instant Pot on the SAUTÉ setting until nearly smoking hot.
2. Add shrimp and sauté 2 minutes before adding onion and garlic. Sauté an additional 2 minutes or until shrimp are mostly pink.
3. Stir in cauliflower rice and continue sautéing 2 minutes.
4. Add white wine and heavy cream and, stirring constantly, bring up to a simmer.
5. Turn off heat, cover, and let stand 4 minutes, uncovering to stir at least once, just until cauliflower is tender.
6. Stir in Parmesan cheese, salt, and pepper before serving topped with chopped parsley.

### Instant Tips

The white wine can be replaced with ½ cup of chicken or vegetable stock and the juice of ½ lemon. This is also really good when garnished with lemon zest, whether you make it with the wine or the stock and lemon juice.

---

**Calories: 385 | Fat: 27g | Protein: 27.5g | Total Carbs: 6g - Fiber: 2g = Net Carbs: 4g**

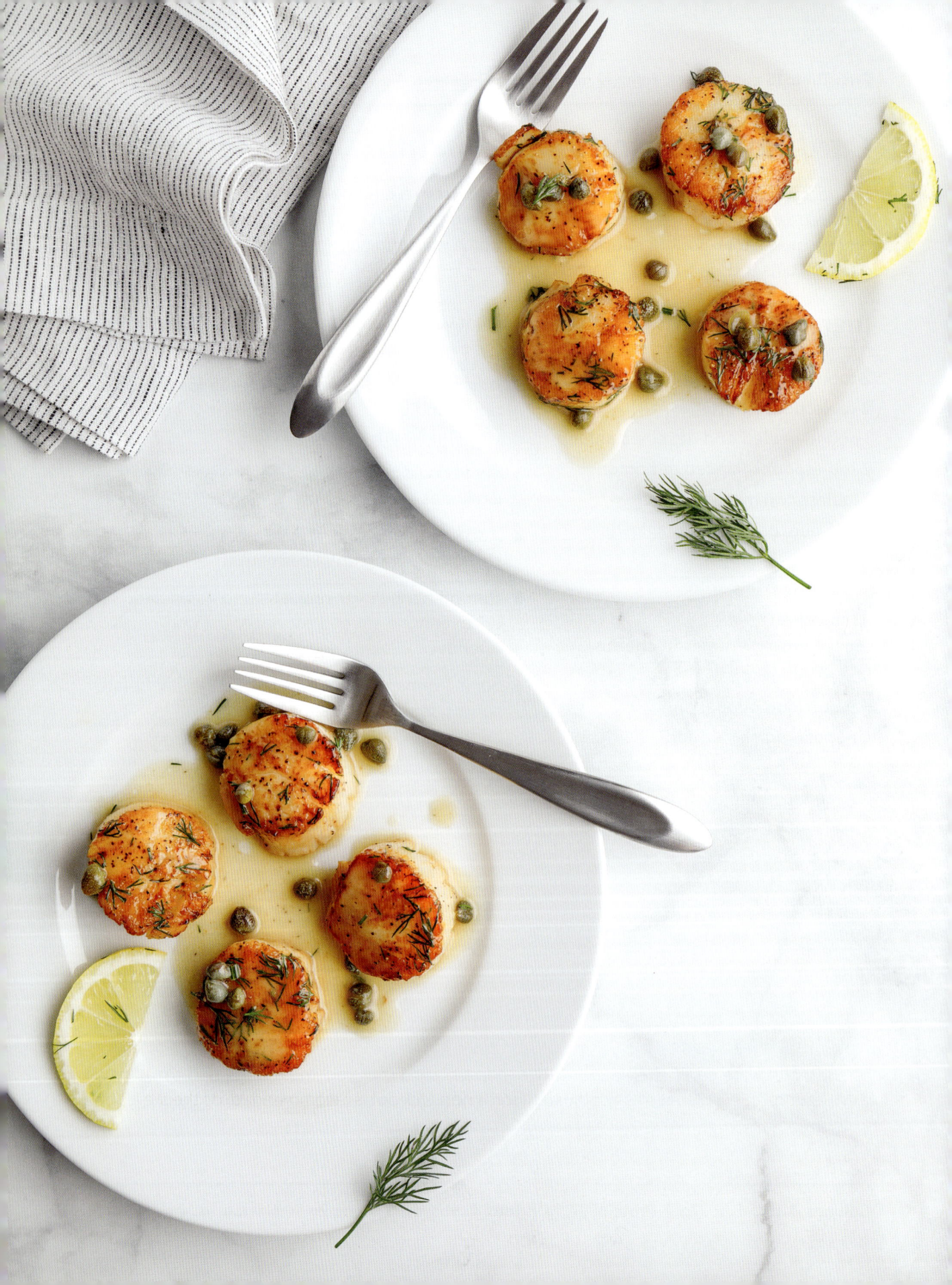

**Prep Time: 10 min | Cook Time: 10 min | Sauté | Serves: 4**

# Scallops with Capers and Dill

Although there aren't many things the Instant Pot cannot excel at, seafood—especially shellfish—can be quite tricky without proper technique. The secret to scallops is simple: a very hot pot and a little patience before flipping.

## Ingredients

1 pound sea (large) scallops
Salt and pepper
3 tablespoons vegetable oil
Juice of ½ lemon
2 tablespoons butter
2 tablespoons capers, drained
2 tablespoons chopped fresh dill

1. For the best results, let scallops stand at room temperature for 10 minutes before cooking. Pat dry and lightly season both sides with salt and pepper.
2. Set the Instant Pot to the SAUTÉ setting and let sit 4 minutes to get hot.
3. Add vegetable oil to the cooker and heat for 2 minutes or until nearly smoking hot.
4. Place the scallops in the cooker and let cook, undisturbed, until they are browned and will release from the cooker, about 3 minutes.
5. Flip and cook the opposite side for 2 minutes.
6. Squeeze lemon juice into the cooker and turn off cooker.
7. Stir in butter, capers, and dill before serving.

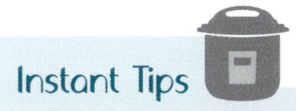

### Instant Tips

To take the stress out of this dish, Instant Pot's nonstick pot is recommended, as the standard pot needs to get very hot to ensure that the scallops do not stick.

**Calories: 245 | Fat: 17g | Protein: 19g | Total Carbs: 4g - Fiber: 0g = Net Carbs: 4g**

Prep Time: 10 min | Cook Time: 8 min | Sauté | Serves: 4

# Spinach with Artichokes

This simple sauté recipe for Spinach "with" Artichokes is not the creamy Spinach "and" Artichokes of the classic dip. This is a lighter dish with olive oil, butter, garlic, and a splash of red wine vinegar that is only topped with a bit of grated Parmesan, instead of swimming in a full cheese sauce.

## Ingredients

1 tablespoon olive oil

2 tablespoons butter

3 tablespoons minced red onion

1 tablespoon minced garlic

1 pound baby spinach

1 (14-ounce) can quartered artichoke hearts, drained

1 tablespoon red wine vinegar

1 teaspoon sugar substitute

Salt and pepper

1/4 cup grated Parmesan cheese

1. Heat olive oil and butter in the Instant Pot on the SAUTÉ setting.

2. Add onion and garlic and sauté 1 minute or until fragrant.

3. Add the spinach and sauté until it cooks down, about 5 minutes.

4. Fold in artichokes, red wine vinegar, and sugar substitute and sauté 1 additional minute to heat the artichokes.

5. Season with salt and pepper to taste before serving topped with Parmesan cheese.

**Instant Tips**

For a creamy cross between creamed spinach and spinach and artichoke dip, simply fold in 6 ounces of herbed cream cheese at the end of cooking.

Calories: 165 | Fat: 12g | Protein: 7g | Total Carbs: 9.5g - Fiber: 4g = Net Carbs: 5.5g

Prep Time: 20 min | Cook Time: 15 min | Sauté | Serves: 6

# Ground Turkey Bolognese

This hearty Italian red sauce with ground turkey is a great choice for any night of the week, as it doesn't take too much effort to prepare and leaves plenty of time to relax, because there's only one pot to clean! You can even stir zucchini noodles right into it before serving.

## Ingredients

3 tablespoons olive oil

1 pound ground turkey

½ cup diced red onion

1 tablespoon minced garlic

1 (15-ounce) can tomato sauce

¼ cup beef stock

¼ cup chopped fresh basil

2 tablespoons tomato paste

2 teaspoons balsamic vinegar

1 teaspoon sugar substitute

1 teaspoon Italian seasoning

½ teaspoon salt

½ teaspoon pepper

¼ teaspoon crushed red pepper flakes

1 tablespoon butter

1. Heat olive oil in the Instant Pot on the SAUTÉ setting.
2. Add the ground turkey and crumble it as it browns.
3. Add the onion and garlic and sauté along with the turkey for 1 minute.
4. Stir in all remaining ingredients except butter and bring up to a simmer. Stirring constantly, let simmer 1 minute.
5. Turn off cooker and let rest 5 minutes (to marry the flavors) before stirring in butter.

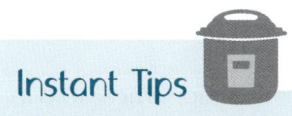

**Instant Tips**

Serve this over spiralized zucchini noodles, spaghetti squash, or ribbons of yellow squash.

Calories: 215 | Fat: 14g | Protein: 16g | Total Carbs: 8g - Fiber: 2g = Net Carbs: 6g

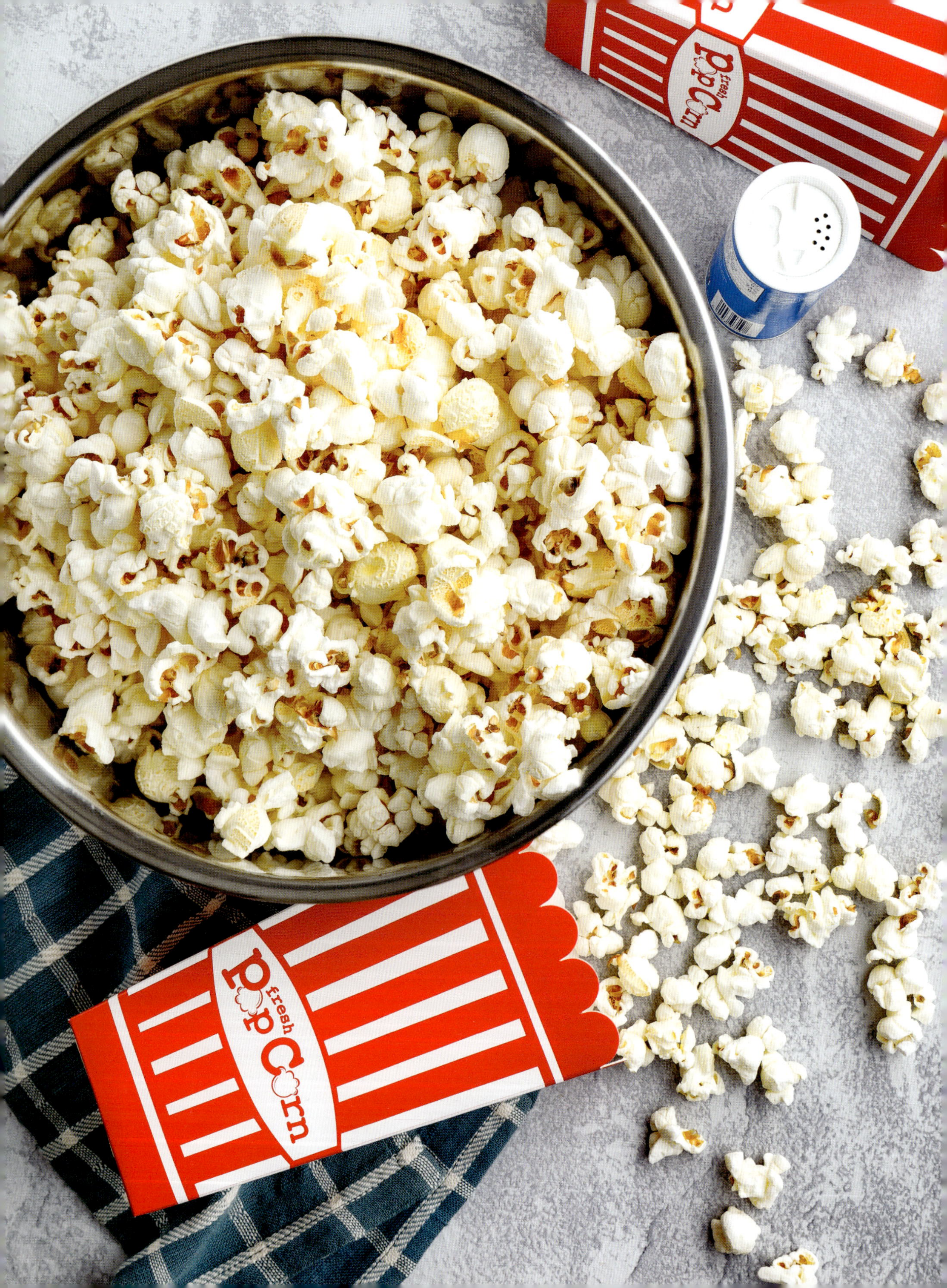
fresh
PopCorn
fresh
PopCorn

Prep Time: 5 min | Cook Time: 6 min | Sauté | Serves: 8

# *Instant Popcorn*

While it isn't suitable for heavily carb-restricted diets such as the ketogenic diet, popcorn can be enjoyed in moderation on looser low-carb lifestyles, especially once you are simply maintaining a weight and not actively trying to lose weight. We've found that making it in the Instant Pot is easier than on the stovetop, as the amount of heat is less likely to cause the popcorn at the bottom to burn. Coconut oil is recommended as it better conducts the heat to get things popping and a 6-quart or larger cooker is a must, or you will need to cut the amounts in half to ensure the corn doesn't overflow.

## Ingredients

**3 tablespoons coconut oil**

**¾ teaspoon salt**

**½ cup popcorn kernels**

## Special Equipment

**Steam rack**

1. Set Instant Pot to SAUTÉ and let the cooker heat up for 5 minutes.
2. Add coconut oil and salt to the cooker and wait until melted and sizzling hot.
3. Using a silicone spatula, swirl the popcorn kernels in the oil to coat.
4. Place a glass lid over the cooker, leaving a small crack for steam to escape (otherwise the popcorn won't be as crisp).
5. In about 3 minutes, the popcorn will start popping. Let pop 2 minutes or until popping has slowed considerably (every 2 seconds or so). Turn off cooker.
6. Using oven mitts, with lid still in place, remove the inner pot from the cooker and shake to move the popcorn around and potentially pop a few more kernels.
7. Serve immediately.

### Instant Tips

We like to salt the oil to ensure it gets onto every kernel, but after popping you can flavor this with additional salt and/or melted butter to taste.

---

Calories: 85 | Fat: 5.5g | Protein: 1g | Total Carbs: 10g - Fiber: 2g = Net Carbs: 8g

Instant Low Carb • 153

Prep Time: 10 min | Cook Time: 8 min | Sauté | Serves: 4

# Cauliflower Fried Rice with Ham

While it may seem strange at first, many combination fried rice dishes (with multiple proteins) include ham, as do Hawaiian versions of the dish. By using ham in place of pork, we can make this a quick sauté that can be made in minutes. As with all of our "rice" recipes, grated cauliflower is used as a substitute for the grain to keep down the carbs.

## Ingredients

- 2 tablespoons vegetable oil
- 12–16 ounces grated cauliflower (cauliflower rice)
- 8 ounces diced ham
- ¼ cup diced red bell pepper
- 3 tablespoons soy sauce
- 2 teaspoons minced garlic
- 2 teaspoons grated fresh ginger
- 1 teaspoon sugar substitute
- ¼ teaspoon pepper
- ¼ cup sliced scallions
- 1 tablespoon sesame oil

1. Heat vegetable oil in the Instant Pot on the SAUTÉ setting.

2. Add cauliflower, ham, and bell pepper and let cook, covered with a glass lid, for 5 minutes, stirring occasionally.

3. Stir in soy sauce, garlic, ginger, sugar substitute, and pepper and sauté an additional 2 minutes or until cauliflower is crisp-tender.

4. Stir in scallions and sesame oil before serving.

### Instant Tips

This can be made easiest with packaged diced ham and a package of riced cauliflower (sold between 12 and 16 ounces). To make your own rice, grate a small head of cauliflower using a cheese grater.

Calories: 195 | Fat: 12g | Protein: 13.5g | Total Carbs: 8.5g - Fiber: 2.5g = Net Carbs: 6g

Prep Time: 20 min | Cook Time: 10 min | Sauté | Serves: 4

# Margherita Chicken with Spaghetti Squash

The fresh flavors in this simple yet delicious sauté of chicken tenderloins and spaghetti squash is reminiscent of a pizza Margherita, which is traditionally made using only three main ingredients—tomato, basil, and cheese—representing the colors of the Italian flag.

## Ingredients

- 3 tablespoons olive oil
- 1 pound chicken tenderloins, chopped
- Salt and pepper
- ¼ cup diced red onion
- 1 tablespoon minced garlic
- 3 cups cooked spaghetti squash
- 1 tomato, diced
- ¼ cup chopped fresh basil
- 2 teaspoons balsamic vinegar
- ⅓ cup grated Parmesan cheese

1. Heat olive oil in the Instant Pot on the SAUTÉ setting.
2. Generously season chicken tenderloins with salt and pepper before adding to the cooker and sautéing 4 minutes or until they begin to lightly brown.
3. Stir in onion and garlic and sauté 2 minutes or until chicken is cooked throughout.
4. Fold spaghetti squash, tomato, basil, and vinegar into the chicken mixture and turn off cooker.
5. Cover and let stand 1 minute to heat the spaghetti squash through.
6. Season with salt and pepper to taste before serving topped with plenty of grated Parmesan cheese.

**Instant Tips**

This is also really good when topped with a large dollop of prepared pesto sauce.

Calories: 265 | Fat: 14.5g | Protein: 27g | Total Carbs: 8g - Fiber: 1.5g = Net Carbs: 6.5g

Instant Low Carb

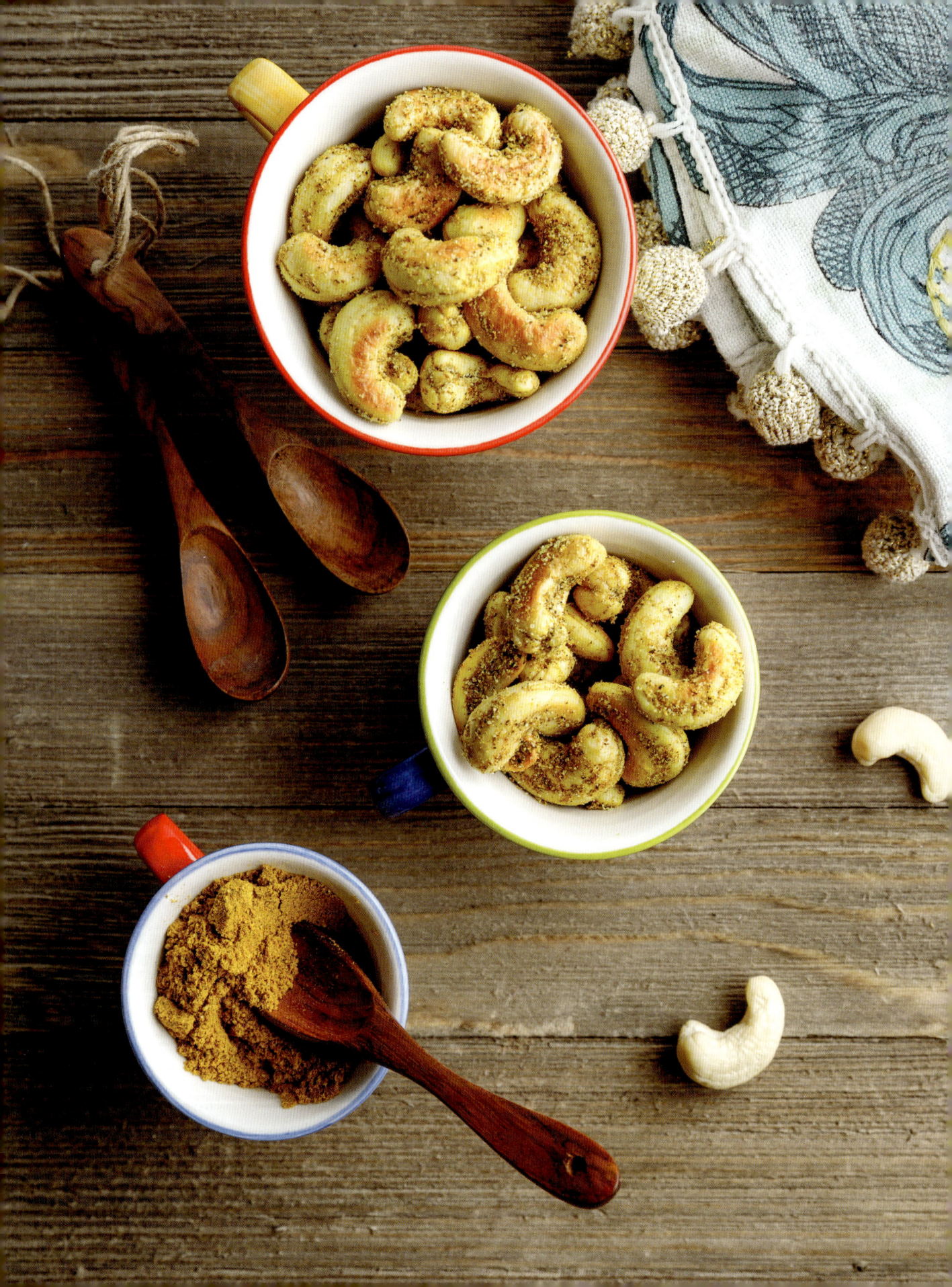

**Prep Time: 5 min | Cook Time: 10 min | Sauté | Serves: 6**

# Indian-Spiced Cashews

The magical warm spice mix of garam masala and curry powder adds a level of complexity to these toasted cashews that is truly unique. A small amount of sugar substitute is added to balance out the earthy spices and give you a bit of that great savory-sweet combination you'd find in a good snack.

## Ingredients

1 tablespoon vegetable oil
1 cup raw cashews
2 teaspoons sugar substitute
½ tablespoon garam masala
½ tablespoon curry powder
½ teaspoon salt

1. Heat vegetable oil in the Instant Pot on the SAUTÉ setting.
2. Stir in cashews, coating them in the oil.
3. Let cashews cook 4 minutes, stirring occasionally, just until they are lightly browned.
4. Stir in sugar substitute, garam masala, curry powder, and salt and cook an additional 2 minutes, stirring constantly.
5. Immediately transfer to a serving dish and let cool 10 minutes before serving.

**Instant Tips**

Garam masala is a dry spice blend often sold in the ethnic foods section but may also be found in the spice section.

**Calories: 130 | Fat: 10g | Protein: 3g | Total Carbs: 6g - Fiber: 1g = Net Carbs: 5g**

**Prep Time:** 10 min | **Cook Time:** 10 min | **Sauté** | **Serves:** 4

# Snap Peas with Crispy Pancetta

Crispy bits of savory pancetta are tossed with sweet snap peas in this easy side dish, made using only a handful of ingredients.

## Ingredients

4 ounces diced pancetta (see tip)

½ pound sugar snap peas, ends snapped

¼ teaspoon garlic powder

¼ teaspoon salt

¼ teaspoon pepper

1 teaspoon lemon zest

1. Heat the pancetta in the Instant Pot on the SAUTÉ setting, cooking until almost crispy.
2. Stir in snap peas, garlic powder, salt, and pepper and sauté 5 minutes or until snap peas are crisp-tender.
3. Stir in lemon zest before serving.

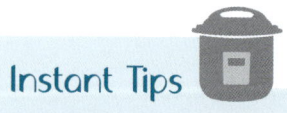

### Instant Tips

Pancetta is an Italian bacon that you can often find pre-diced near the gourmet cheeses in the deli section. Regular diced bacon can be substituted in a pinch.

**Calories:** 130 | **Fat:** 9g | **Protein:** 5g | **Total Carbs:** 4.5g - **Fiber:** 1.5g = **Net Carbs:** 3g

**Prep Time: 15 min | Cook Time: 15 min | Sauté | Serves: 4**

# Cheesy Ground Beef Skillet

There really isn't a need for noodles in this one-pot "skillet" meal that tastes like a deconstructed cheeseburger. Chopped yellow squash helps fill the dish out in place of any high-carb starches.

## Ingredients

1 tablespoon vegetable oil
1 pound ground beef
4 ounces sliced mushrooms
¼ cup diced red onion
2 cups chopped yellow squash
½ cup beef broth
1 teaspoon Worcestershire sauce
1 teaspoon celery salt
½ teaspoon pepper
½ teaspoon dried oregano
¼ teaspoon garlic powder
2 ounces cream cheese
1 cup shredded sharp Cheddar cheese

1. Heat vegetable oil in the Instant Pot on the SAUTÉ setting.
2. Add the ground beef and crumble it as it browns.
3. Add the mushrooms and onion and sauté along with the beef for 2 minutes. Drain excess grease.
4. Stir in all remaining ingredients except cream cheese and Cheddar cheese and bring up to a simmer.
5. Cover with a glass lid and let cook 4 minutes or until squash is tender.
6. Turn off cooker and stir in cream cheese and Cheddar cheese before serving.

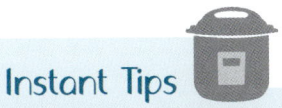

**Instant Tips**

The sharper the Cheddar cheese, the more flavor this will have, which is a good reason to shred your own extra-sharp cheese.

Calories: 460 | Fat: 34.5g | Protein: 30g | Total Carbs: 6.5g - Fiber: 1g = Net Carbs: 5.5g

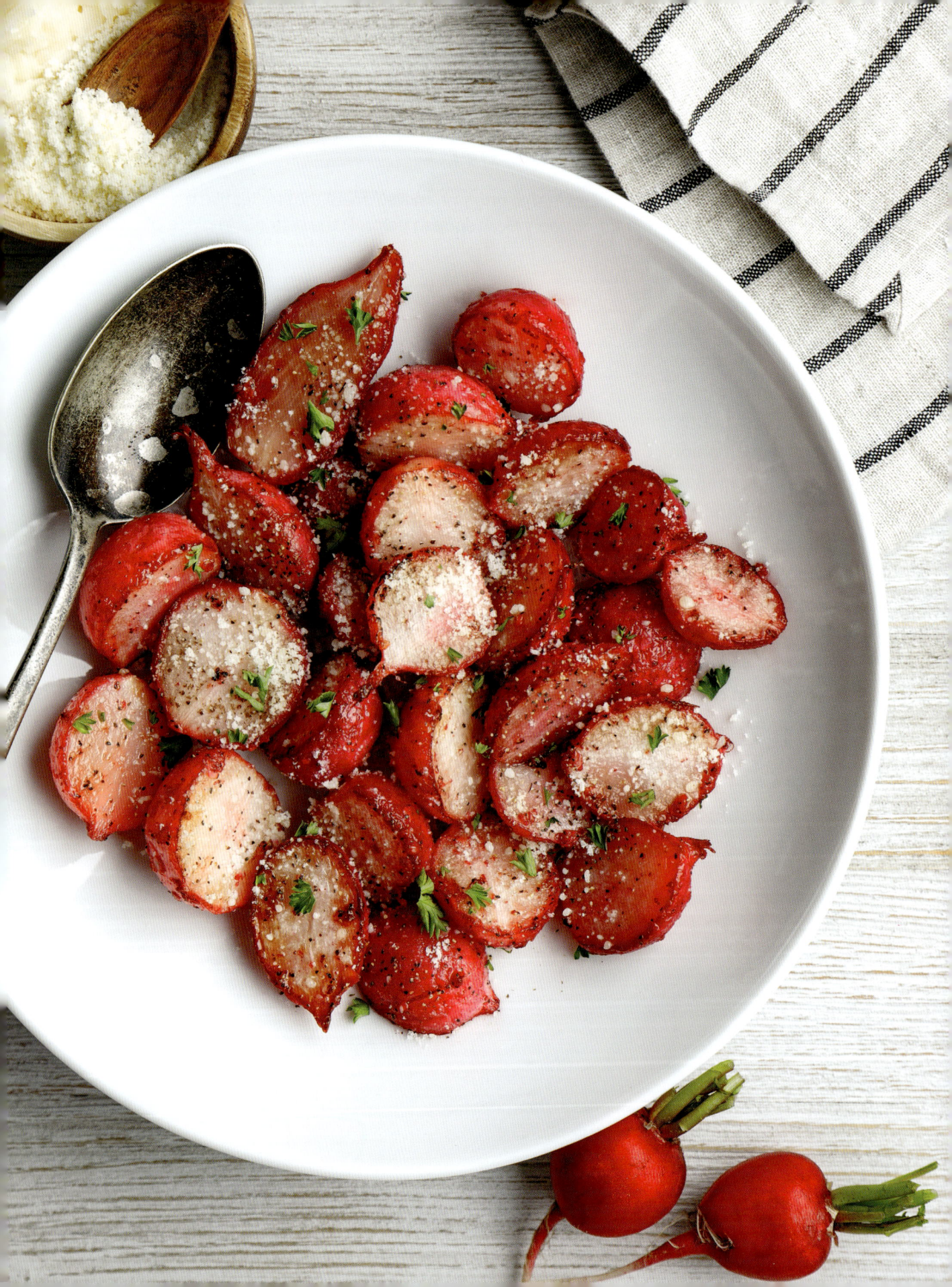

Prep Time: 10 min | Cook Time: 10 min | Sauté | Serves: 4

# Red Bliss Radishes

We've said it before, but we'll say it again: radishes are amazing! Here, they're the perfect stand-in for red bliss potatoes, presenting the same subtle earthiness and a surprisingly similar texture. To complete their transformation into low-carb potatoes, they are sautéed in butter and tossed with garlic, Parmesan cheese, and parsley.

## Ingredients

- 2 tablespoons vegetable oil
- 1 tablespoon butter
- 1 pound radishes, trimmed and halved
- ¼ teaspoon salt
- ¼ teaspoon pepper
- ¼ teaspoon onion powder
- 2 teaspoons minced garlic
- ¼ cup grated Parmesan cheese
- 2 tablespoons chopped fresh parsley

1. Heat vegetable oil and butter in the Instant Pot on the SAUTÉ setting.
2. Add radishes, salt, pepper, and onion powder and sauté until radishes begin to brown, about 8 minutes.
3. Add garlic and continue sautéing 1 additional minute or until radishes are fork-tender.
4. Toss radishes in Parmesan cheese and parsley just before serving.

### Instant Tips

Most stores sell trimmed radishes in a 1-pound bag near the carrots. This is the most convenient way to make this recipe, though you may still have to trim the tops of a few radishes in the bag.

Calories: 135 | Fat: 12g | Protein: 4g | Total Carbs: 4g - Fiber: 2g = Net Carbs: 2g

Instant Low Carb

# Chapter 7: Holiday Cooking

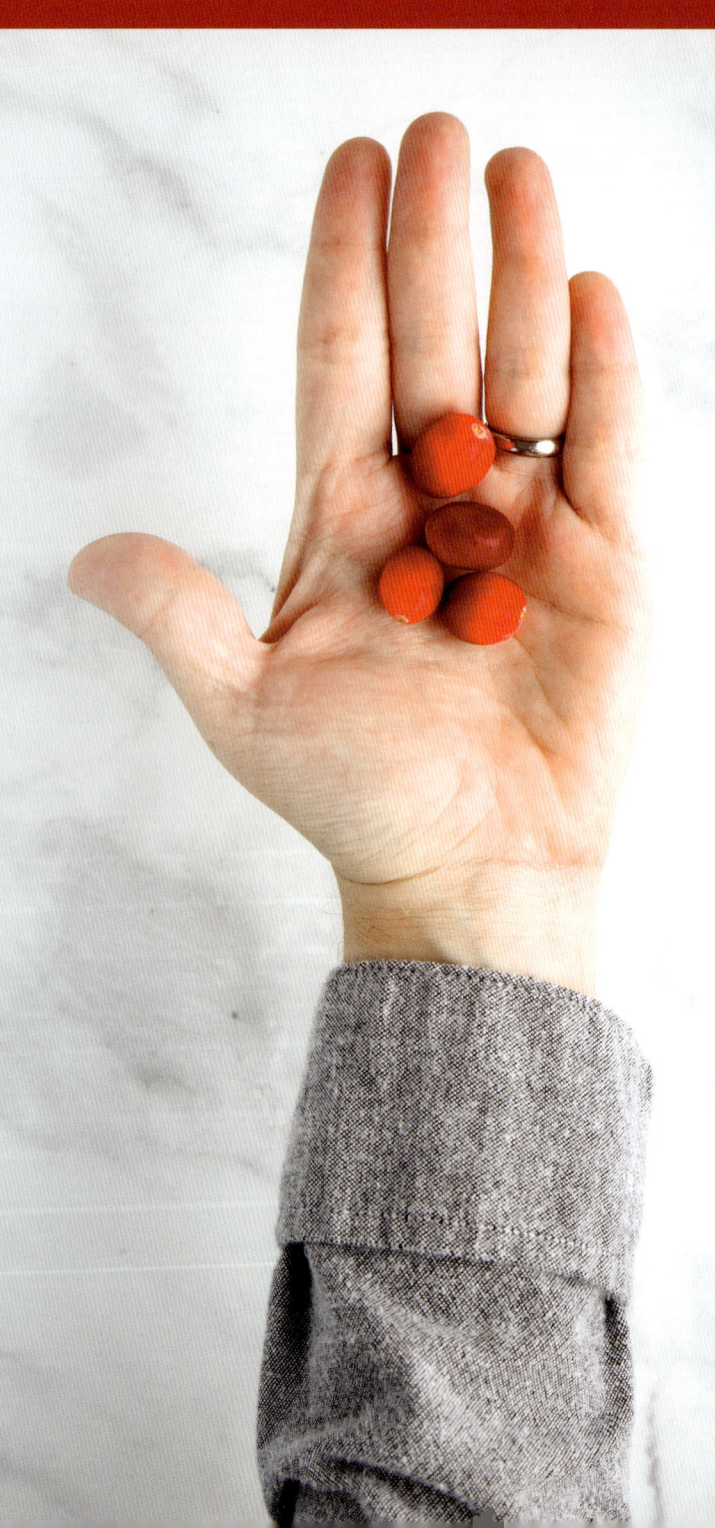

*recipes in this chapter...*

*Secret Message #7: We somehow ended up with 4 extra pounds of fresh cranberries in our freezer during the making of this book.*

**Tender Turkey Breast**, 165

**Cranberry Walnut Chutney**, 167

**Holiday Ham**, 168

**Sausage Stuffing**, 169

**Butternut Squash Soup**, 171

**Cinnamon and Sage Pork Tenderloin**, 172

**Zesty Kale with Pistachios**, 173

**Casserole-Style Green Beans**, 175

**Maple Pecan Sprouts**, 176

**Eggnog Cake with Bourbon Sauce**, 177

**Pumpkin Pie**, 179

Holidays

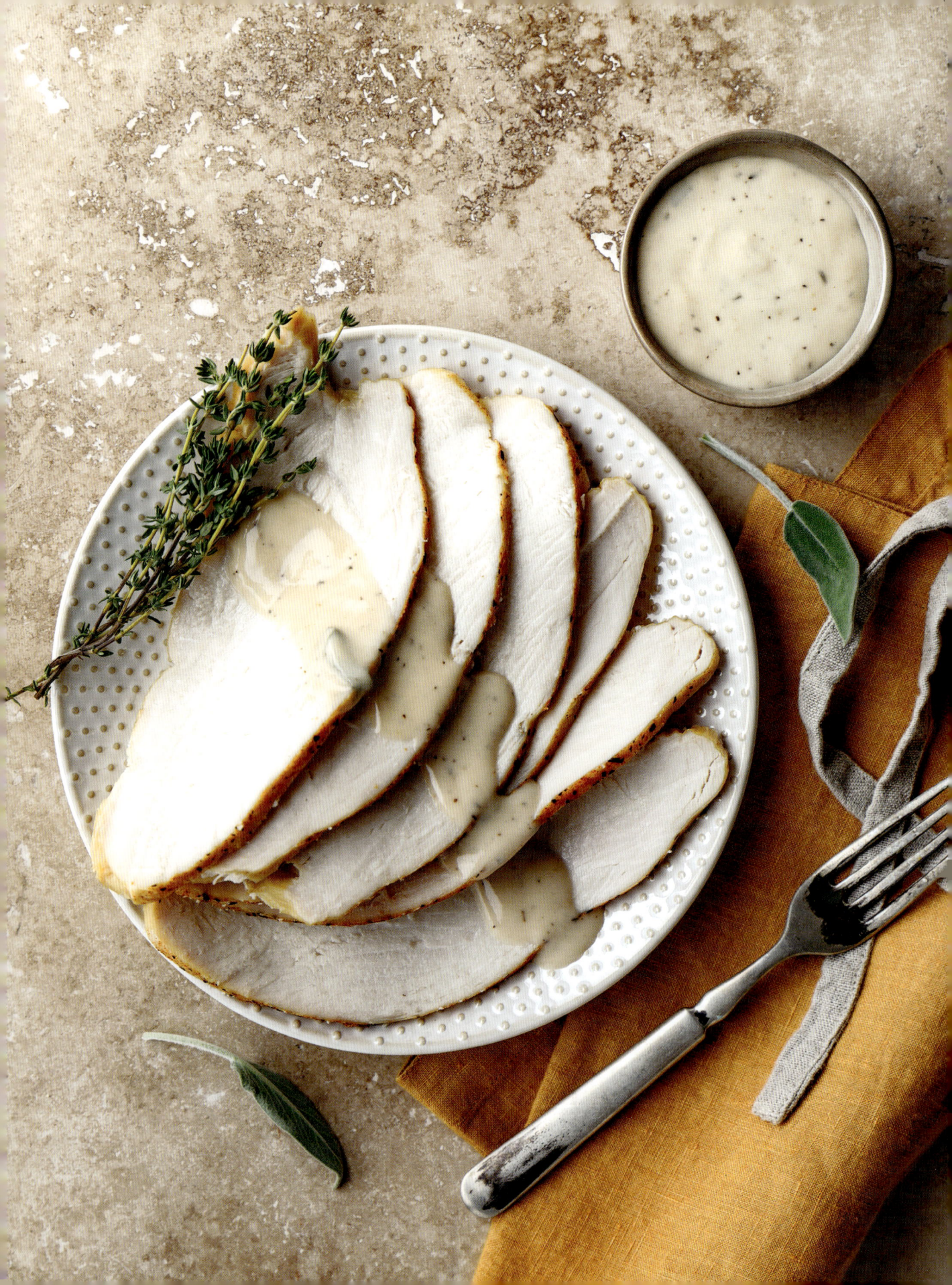

Prep Time: 5 min | High Pressure: 35 min | Natural Release: 15 min | Serves: 10

# Tender Turkey Breast

There is no need to worry about this turkey drying out, as the Instant Pot locks in the moisture during the cooking process, guaranteeing great results. And simply because gravy is a must for the holidays, we've included a foolproof recipe for a creamy pan gravy with sage.

## Ingredients

2 cups chicken stock

1 bone-in fresh turkey breast (about 7 pounds)

2 tablespoons butter, melted

1 teaspoon salt

3/4 teaspoon paprika

1/2 teaspoon poultry seasoning

1/2 teaspoon pepper

1/4 teaspoon dried thyme

1/4 teaspoon garlic powder

1/4 teaspoon onion powder

## Quick Gravy

1 cup heavy cream

3 leaves fresh sage, chopped

2 tablespoons butter

Salt and pepper

## Special Equipment

Steam rack

1. Pour chicken stock in Instant Pot and place steam rack over top.

2. If your turkey breast came with a gravy packet, locate the packet and discard before cooking.

3. Rub melted butter over the entire surface of the turkey breast. For even more flavor, loosen skin and rub the butter under the skin as well.

4. Combine all spices to create a spice rub. Rub the spice rub over the entire surface of the turkey breast. Place seasoned turkey breast on the steam rack in the cooker.

5. Lock lid in place and seal pressure release vent. Set cooker to HIGH pressure for 35 minutes.

6. Let pressure release naturally for 15 minutes before opening the vent to let out remaining pressure. Remove turkey breast from cooker, cover with aluminum foil, and let rest 10 minutes before carving to serve.

**Quick Gravy:** Create a Quick Gravy (as the turkey rests) by discarding all but 1 1/4 cups of the liquid from the cooker. Set cooker to SAUTÉ and let simmer until liquid has reduced by about 1/2. Stir in heavy cream and sage and let simmer 3 additional minutes. Turn off heat and stir in butter before seasoning with salt and pepper to taste.

### Instant Tips

For more color and crispy skin, place the cooked turkey breast under the broiler for 3 to 4 minutes, just until lightly browned.

Calories: 520 | Fat: 20g | Protein: 79g | Total Carbs: 0g - Fiber: 0g = Net Carbs: 0g

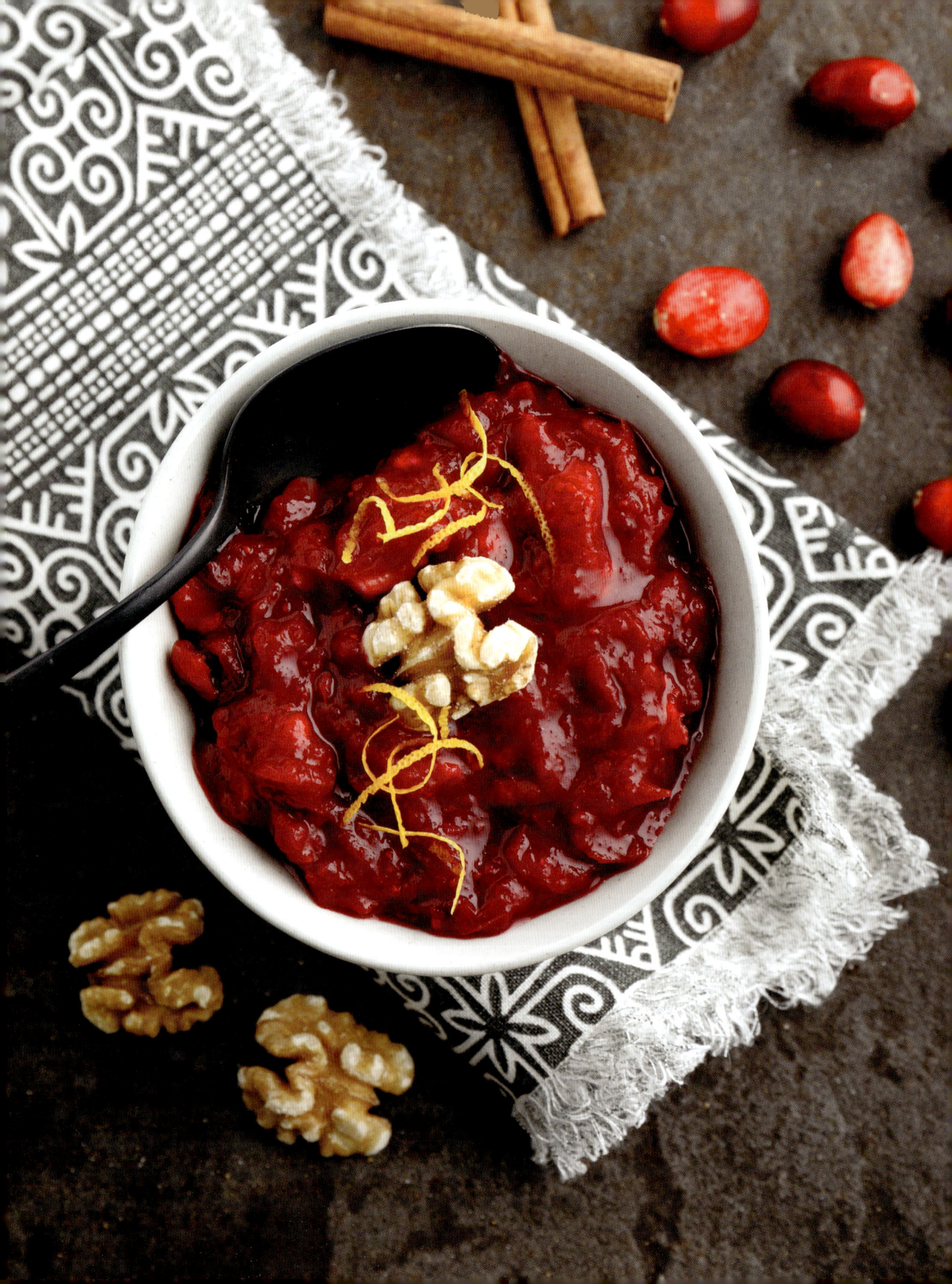

**Prep Time: 5 min | High Pressure: 2 min | Natural Release: 5 min | Serves: 8**

# Cranberry Walnut Chutney

Everyone knows that a traditional Thanksgiving spread isn't quite complete without a bowl of cranberry sauce somewhere on the table. This chutney not only fills that requirement, it's also easy to make and isn't loaded with the sugar of those unmentionable can-shaped logs of jelly. We always buy an extra bag or two of fresh cranberries when they're in season, then store them in the freezer so that we can enjoy cranberry chutney throughout the year.

## Ingredients

12 ounces fresh cranberries
1 cup sugar substitute
½ cup water
2 teaspoons orange zest
1 teaspoon vegetable oil
¼ teaspoon ground cinnamon
½ cup chopped walnuts

1. Add all ingredients except walnuts to the Instant Pot and stir to combine.
2. Lock lid in place and seal pressure release vent. Set cooker to HIGH pressure for 2 minutes.
3. Let pressure release naturally for 5 minutes before carefully opening the vent to let out remaining pressure.
4. Stir walnuts into the chutney before serving. For the thickest texture, serve chilled.

**Holidays**

### Instant Tips

To thicken the chutney even further, after pressure cooking, set cooker to SAUTÉ and bring up to a simmer. Stirring constantly, let simmer until slightly thickened.

**Calories: 75 | Fat: 5.5g | Protein: 1g | Total Carbs: 8.5g - Fiber: 2g = Net Carbs: 6.5g**

Instant Low Carb • 167

Prep Time: 5 min | High Pressure: 15 min | Natural Release: 10 min | Serves: 12

# Holiday Ham

The whole ham, just the way it was meant to be, heated through in just under half an hour—giving you more time to do the things that matter most, like spending it with family, friends, and pets.

## Ingredients

1 small bone-in ham (about 6 pounds)
2 tablespoons sugar substitute
1 tablespoon butter, melted
1 tablespoon Dijon mustard
¼ teaspoon maple extract
¼ teaspoon ground cloves
½ cup water

1. For the best results, let ham sit at room temperature for 30 minutes before preparing.
2. In a small bowl, combine the sugar substitute, butter, Dijon, maple extract, and cloves.
3. Rub the Dijon mixture over the entire surface of the ham.
4. Place the ham directly into the cooker, cut-side down. Pour in water.
5. Lock lid in place and seal pressure release vent. Set cooker to HIGH pressure for 15 minutes.
6. Let pressure release naturally for 10 minutes before opening vent to release any remaining pressure.
7. Let rest 5 minutes before slicing to serve.

### Instant Tips

Look for a standard ham, sometimes labeled "semi-boneless." You don't want anything fancy and spiral sliced, as those often contain a ton of added sugar.

Calories: 335 | Fat: 22g | Protein: 32g | Total Carbs: 0.5g - Fiber: 0g = Net Carbs: 0.5g

Prep Time: 15 min | High Pressure: 0 min | Quick Release | Serves: 4

# Sausage Stuffing

Over the years, we've found that breadcrumbs aren't necessary when it comes to making this traditional holiday side from scratch, as it really is the herbs that make a good stuffing so special.

## Ingredients

1 tablespoon vegetable oil
1 pound ground pork sausage
1 cup chopped mushrooms
3/4 cup diced celery
1/2 cup diced yellow onion
2 teaspoons minced garlic
1/3 cup chicken stock
1 tablespoon chopped fresh sage
2 teaspoons sugar substitute
1/2 teaspoon dried rosemary
1/2 teaspoon salt
1/4 teaspoon pepper
1 tablespoon butter

1. Heat vegetable oil in the Instant Pot on the SAUTÉ setting.
2. Add the sausage and crumble it as it browns. Drain excess grease.
3. Add the mushrooms, celery, onion, and garlic and sauté along with the sausage for 1 minute.
4. Stir in chicken stock, sage, sugar substitute, rosemary, salt, and pepper.
5. Lock lid in place and seal pressure release vent. Set cooker to HIGH pressure for 0 minutes.
6. Carefully open vent to quickly release the pressure.
7. Stir in butter before serving with a slotted spoon.

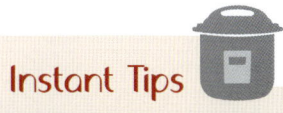

**Instant Tips**
The leftovers of this stuffing are great when served alongside eggs as a breakfast hash.

Calories: 315 | Fat: 23g | Protein: 21.5g | Total Carbs: 4.5g - Fiber: 1g = Net Carbs: 3.5g

Instant Low Carb

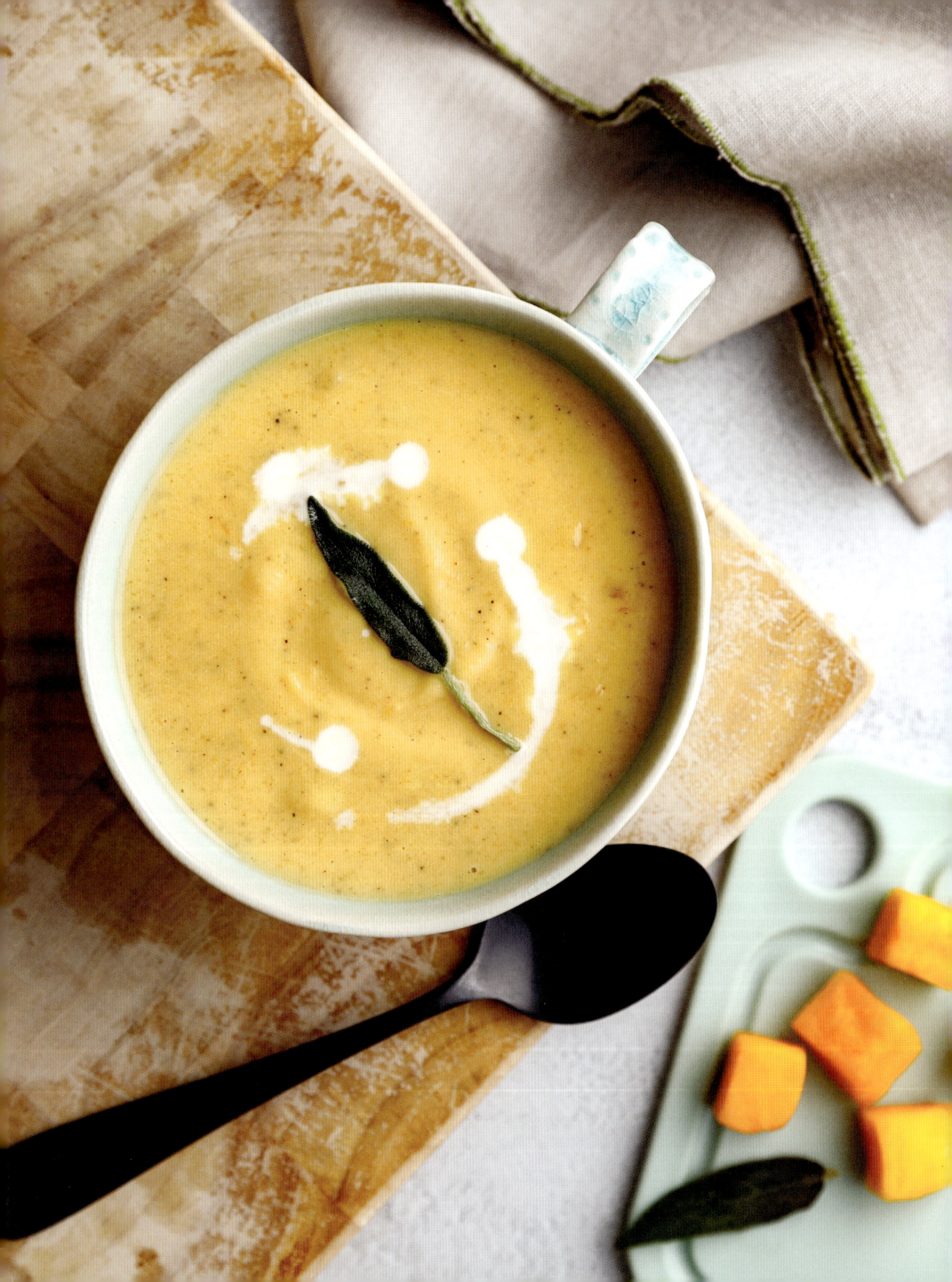

Prep Time: 10 min | High Pressure: 3 min | Quick Release | Serves: 6

# Butternut Squash Soup

Butternut squash, like most winter squash, is relatively high in carbs but has a pretty low "glycemic load," which just means that it may not spike blood sugar as much as other foods. That said, due to the carbs, we only recommend it in smaller portions, which is one of the reasons why we've secretly bulked up this creamy soup by using cauliflower alongside less squash than is ordinarily needed.

## Ingredients

- 1 (10-ounce) bag frozen cubed butternut squash
- 2 cups chopped cauliflower
- 2 cups chicken stock
- 1/2 cup diced yellow onion
- 2 tablespoons sugar substitute
- 1 tablespoon chopped fresh sage
- 1/2 teaspoon dried thyme
- 1/2 teaspoon salt
- 1/2 teaspoon pepper
- 1/4 teaspoon onion powder
- 1/4 teaspoon ground nutmeg
- 1/2 cup heavy cream

1. Place all ingredients except heavy cream in the Instant Pot and toss to combine.
2. Lock lid in place and seal pressure release vent. Set cooker to HIGH pressure for 3 minutes.
3. Carefully open vent to quickly release the pressure.
4. Use an immersion blender to fully purée the soup until smooth. This can also be done by carefully transferring to a food processor or blender.
5. Stir in heavy cream before serving.

### Instant Tips

If the soup has cooled by the time you've added the heavy cream, simply set the cooker to SAUTÉ and bring up to a simmer.

Calories: 105 | Fat: 8g | Protein: 2g | Total Carbs: 8.5g - Fiber: 2g = Net Carbs: 6.5g

Prep Time: 10 min | High Pressure: 2 min | Natural Release: 10 min | Serves: 6

# Cinnamon and Sage Pork Tenderloin

Tender sliced pork is rubbed with an earthy autumn-spice blend of cinnamon and allspice but made even more aromatic with fresh sage, orange zest, and a dash of sherry wine. It's easier to prepare and a nice change of pace from your typical holiday turkey.

## Ingredients

1 cup chicken stock
Zest of 1 orange
2 tablespoons chopped fresh sage
1 tablespoon sherry cooking wine
1 tablespoon vegetable oil
2 teaspoons sugar substitute
1 teaspoon ground cinnamon
1 teaspoon salt
3/4 teaspoon pepper
1/2 teaspoon allspice
2 pork tenderloins

### Special Equipment
Steam rack

1. Pour chicken stock into Instant Pot and place a steam rack over top.
2. In a small bowl, combine the orange zest, sage, sherry, vegetable oil, sugar substitute, cinnamon, salt, pepper, and allspice.
3. Rub the spice mixture into all sides of each pork tenderloin before placing on the steam rack in the cooker.
4. Lock lid in place and seal pressure release vent. Set cooker to HIGH pressure for 2 minutes.
5. Let pressure release naturally for 10 minutes before opening vent to release any remaining pressure.
6. Use a meat thermometer to check for doneness. As long as it reads 145° F or above, the pork is done. If pork is under 145° F, secure the cooker's lid without turning it on and let the residual heat continue cooking the pork for 2 minutes at a time, just until it reaches temperature.
7. Let pork rest 10 minutes before slicing to serve.

**Instant Tips**

For better color, you can place the pork tenderloins under the broiler for just 2 minutes after pressure cooking but not any longer, as they cook fast!

Calories: 320 | Fat: 7.5g | Protein: 56g | Total Carbs: 1g - Fiber: 0g = Net Carbs: 1g

**Prep Time:** 10 min  |  **High Pressure:** 3 min  |  **Quick Release**  |  **Serves:** 6

# Zesty Kale with Pistachios

Raw kale can be a bit bitter, but it cooks up nice and sweet in this simple recipe with orange zest and chopped pistachios for crunch. Kale is a bit high in natural carbs, but they're from a very healthy source. That said, if you are watching your carbs closely, we recommend the small portion size of this recipe (6 servings from the full dish).

## Ingredients

- 1 tablespoon vegetable oil
- ½ cup diced yellow onion
- 1 pound chopped kale
- ½ cup water
- 2 teaspoons sugar substitute
- ½ teaspoon salt
- ¼ teaspoon pepper
- Zest of 1 small orange, divided
- ⅓ cup chopped pistachios
- 1 tablespoon butter

1. Heat vegetable oil in the Instant Pot on the SAUTÉ setting.
2. Add the onion and sauté 4 minutes or until onions begin to cook down.
3. Stir in kale, water, sugar substitute, salt, pepper, and ½ of the orange zest.
4. Lock lid in place and seal pressure release vent. Set cooker to HIGH pressure for 3 minutes.
5. Carefully open vent to quickly release the pressure.
6. Stir in chopped pistachios, butter, and the remaining ½ of the orange zest before serving.

**Holidays**

### Instant Tips

This is also great with chopped walnuts or pecans, as we know that shelled pistachios can be on the pricey side.

**Calories:** 120  |  **Fat:** 7.5g  |  **Protein:** 4g  |  **Total Carbs:** 11g  -  **Fiber:** 3g  =  **Net Carbs:** 8g

Instant Low Carb • 173

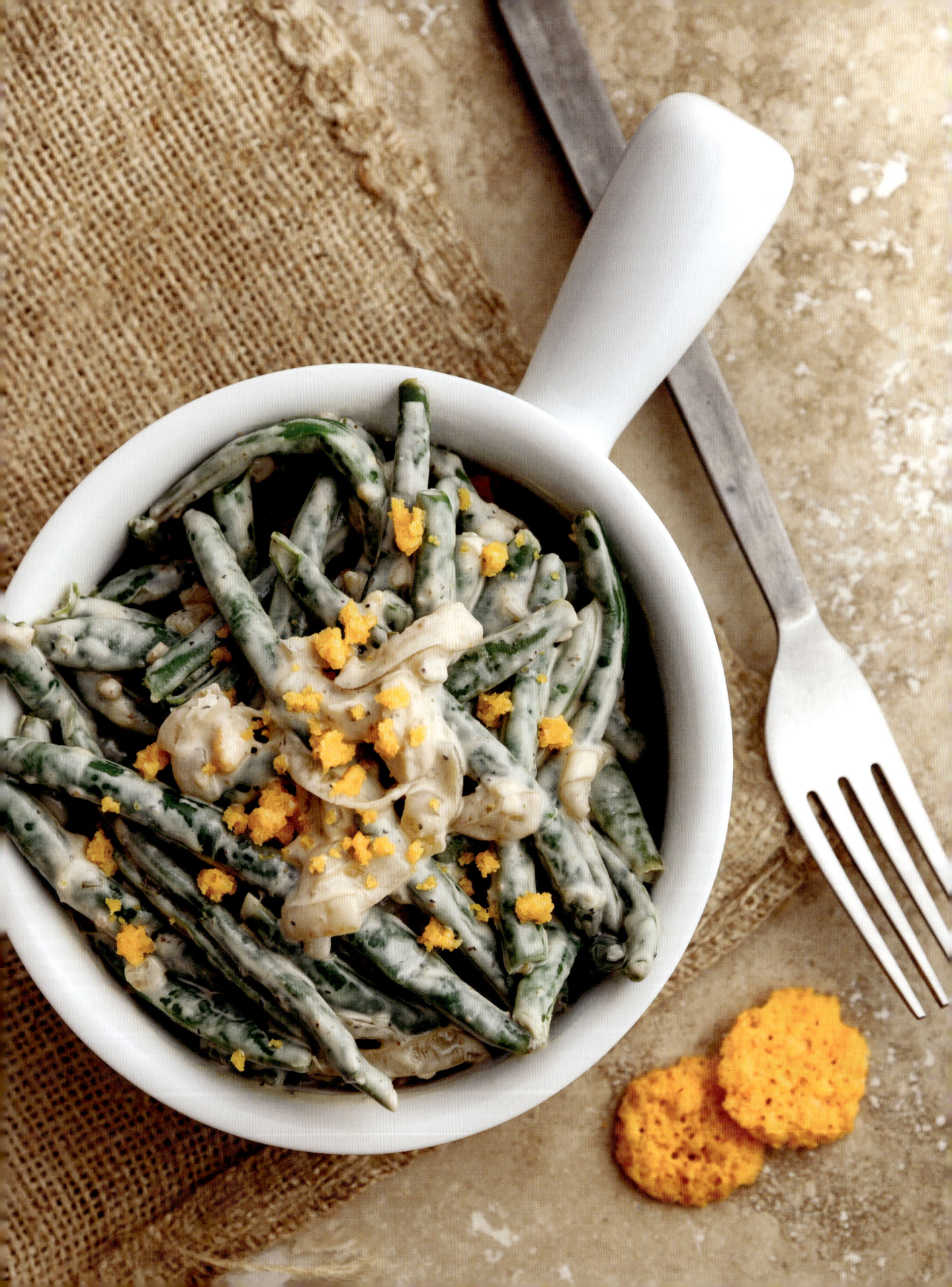

Prep Time: 10 min | High Pressure: 0 min | Quick Release | Serves: 4

# Casserole-Style Green Beans

Green vegetables like this are extremely easy to overcook under pressure, but the secret is a 0-minute cook time that only lets the cooker come up to pressure before stopping. We then stir in herbed cream cheese spread to make a creamy sauce without having to use a ton of ingredients.

## Ingredients

- 1 tablespoon butter
- 1/4 yellow onion, thinly sliced
- 2 teaspoons minced garlic
- 2/3 cup beef stock
- 1 pound green beans, trimmed
- 4 ounces herbed cream cheese
- Salt and pepper
- Crushed cheese crackers, optional (see tip)

1. Heat butter in the Instant Pot on the SAUTÉ setting.
2. Place onion and garlic in the cooker and sauté until onions are translucent and garlic is beginning to brown, about 5 minutes.
3. Add beef stock and green beans to the cooker and toss to combine.
4. Lock lid in place and seal pressure release vent. Set cooker to HIGH pressure for 0 minutes.
5. Carefully open vent to quickly release the pressure.
6. Drain 3/4 of the liquid from the cooker. Stir in herbed cream cheese and season with salt and pepper to taste. If this cools the green beans too much, simply set the cooker to SAUTÉ for 1 minute, stirring constantly, just until warmed. Serve topped with crushed cheese crackers, if desired.

### Instant Tips

For a bit of crunch, we like to top this with 100% cheese crackers, which you can now find in most stores, sold in pouches (not cracker boxes) in the produce, gluten-free, or healthy snack foods section. Check the ingredients for crackers that are entirely made from cheese.

Calories: 170 | Fat: 12g | Protein: 4g | Total Carbs: 11.5g - Fiber: 4g = Net Carbs: 7.5g

Instant Low Carb • 175

Prep Time: 10 min | High Pressure: 1 min | Quick Release | Serves: 4

# Maple Pecan Sprouts

These brussels sprouts are in a light and buttery maple sauce, tossed with pecans for a bit of a crunch. Though they are considered a winter vegetable, we'll eat this recipe all year round!

## Ingredients

½ cup vegetable stock
½ teaspoon maple extract
1 pound brussels sprouts, halved
2 tablespoons butter
½ cup pecan halves or pieces
Salt and pepper

## Special Equipment

Steam basket

1. Pour vegetable stock and maple extract in the Instant Pot and place a steam basket over top.
2. Place brussels sprouts in steam basket.
3. Lock lid in place and seal pressure release vent. Set cooker to HIGH pressure for 1 minute.
4. Carefully open vent to quickly release the pressure. Carefully remove steam basket.
5. Drain ¾ of the liquid from the cooker before stirring in butter and pecans.
6. Toss cooked brussels sprouts in the butter sauce with pecans before seasoning with a generous amount of salt and pepper to taste.

*Holidays*

### Instant Tips

This is also great with cooked and crumbled bacon added at the same time you add the pecans.

Calories: 195 | Fat: 16g | Protein: 5g | Total Carbs: 11.5g - Fiber: 5g = Net Carbs: 6.5g

Prep Time: 20 min | High Pressure: 45 min | Natural Release: 10 min | Serves: 8

# Eggnog Cake with Bourbon Sauce

This light and creamy bar cake has the essence of eggnog and is topped with a drizzle of spiked bourbon syrup that will leave you feeling all warm and fuzzy inside, regardless of whether you're near a roaring fireplace.

## Ingredients

Nonstick cooking spray
1 ½ cups almond flour
⅔ cup sugar substitute
1 ½ teaspoons baking powder
½ teaspoon ground nutmeg
¼ teaspoon ground cinnamon
4 large egg whites
4 tablespoons butter, melted
¼ cup heavy cream
1 ½ teaspoons vanilla extract

### Bourbon Sauce

2 tablespoons bourbon whiskey
¼ cup heavy cream
3 tablespoons sugar substitute
¼ teaspoon vanilla extract

### Special Equipment

6.5-inch loaf pan
Steam rack

1. Pour 1 cup of water into the Instant Pot. Spray a 6.5-inch loaf pan with nonstick cooking spray.

2. In a mixing bowl, combine almond flour, sugar substitute, baking powder, nutmeg, and cinnamon.

3. In a separate mixing bowl, whisk together egg whites, butter, heavy cream, and vanilla extract until egg whites are frothy. Fold the wet ingredients into the dry ingredients to create a cake batter.

4. Spread the batter into the prepared loaf pan and tap against the counter to even out the top. Wrap bottom and all sides of the loaf pan in aluminum foil to prevent any water from seeping in. Place wrapped loaf pan on steam rack and carefully lower into the water bath in the Instant Pot.

5. Lock lid in place and seal pressure release vent. Set cooker to HIGH pressure for 45 minutes.

6. Let pressure release naturally for 10 minutes before opening the vent to let out any remaining pressure.

7. Let cool on counter for at least 30 minutes before refrigerating at least 2 hours.

**Bourbon Sauce:** In a small saucepan over medium heat, whisk together all Bourbon Sauce ingredients and bring up to a simmer. Whisking occasionally, let simmer 2 minutes before serving warm, drizzled sparingly over slices of the cake.

### Instant Tips

The alcohol in the Bourbon Sauce will cook out as it simmers, but you also can skip the sauce entirely if the flavor of bourbon isn't desired.

---

Calories: 260 | Fat: 22g | Protein: 6.5g | Total Carbs: 7.5g - Fiber: 2.5g = Net Carbs: 5g

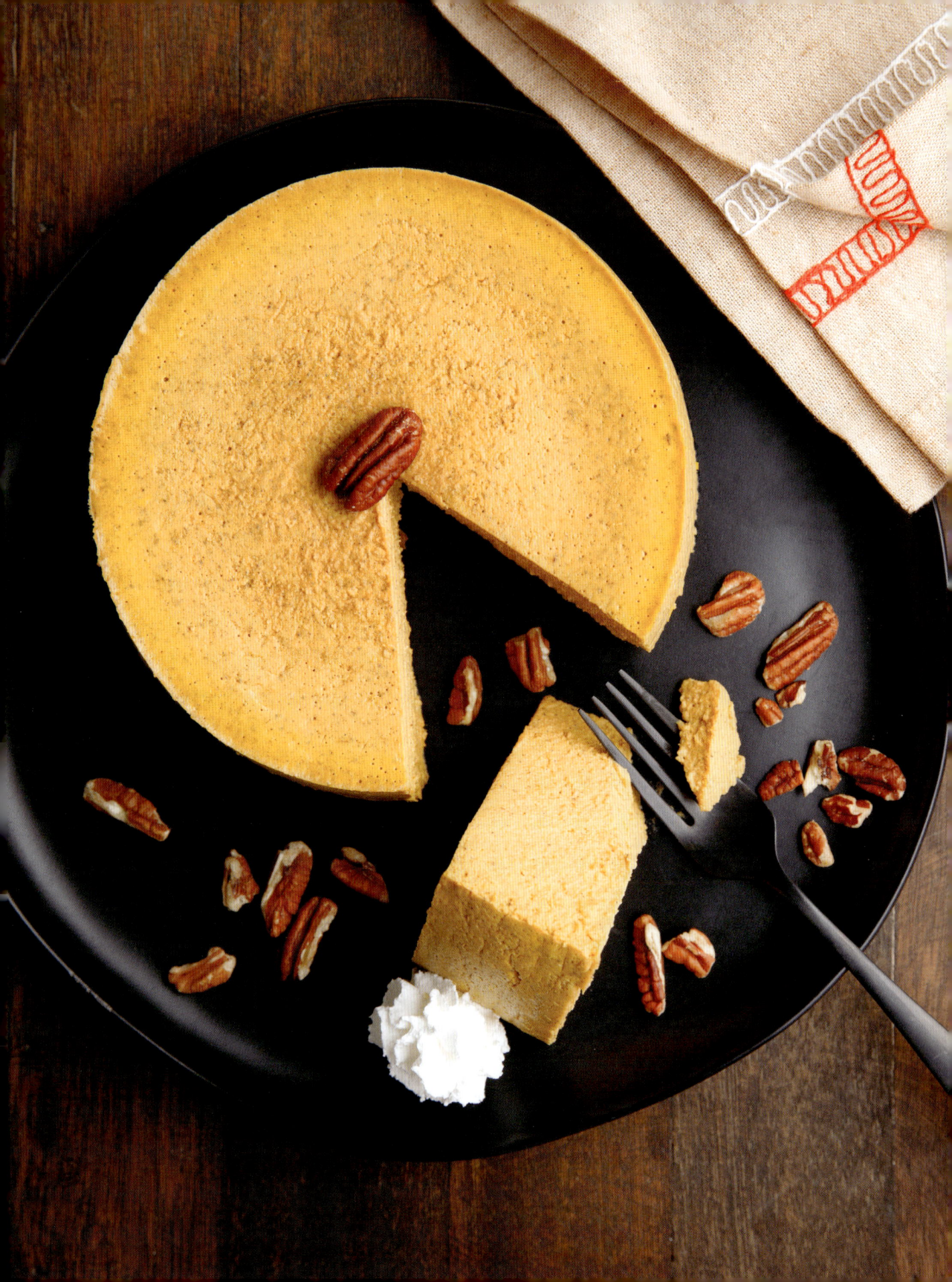

Prep Time: 10 min | High Pressure: 60 min | Natural Release: 15 min | Serves: 8

# Pumpkin Pie

When it comes to festive desserts, there really is nothing humbler or more heartwarming than good ol' pumpkin pie. Thankfully stores now sell cans of sugar-free whipped cream, which we highly recommend as a topping for this pie, though we find whipping our own is usually worth the extra effort.

## Ingredients

Nonstick cooking spray
1 (15-ounce) can 100% pure pumpkin
²/₃ cup heavy cream
²/₃ cup sugar substitute
3 large eggs
1 large egg yolk
1 tablespoon pumpkin pie spice
¼ teaspoon vanilla extract

## Special Equipment

7-inch springform pan
Steam rack

1. Pour 1 cup of water into the Instant Pot. Spray a 7-inch springform pan with nonstick cooking spray.
2. In a mixing bowl, whisk all remaining ingredients until smooth and combined.
3. Pour the batter into the prepared cake pan and tap against the counter to remove any air bubbles. Tightly wrap the bottom and top of the pan to ensure it is watertight before placing on steam rack. Carefully lower into the water bath in the Instant Pot.
4. Lock lid in place and seal pressure release vent. Set cooker to HIGH pressure for 60 minutes.
5. Let pressure release naturally for 15 minutes before opening vent to release any remaining pressure.
6. Cool on counter for at least 30 minutes, then chill at least 4 hours before slicing to serve.

### Instant Tips

When we make pumpkin pie in the oven, we typically create a crust out of chopped pecans, but they get soggy when made under pressure. To get that same crunch, we simply sprinkle chopped pecans over top the sliced pie.

Calories: 125 | Fat: 10.5g | Protein: 3g | Total Carbs: 7g - Fiber: 1.5g = Net Carbs: 5.5g

*Chapter 8*

# Sides

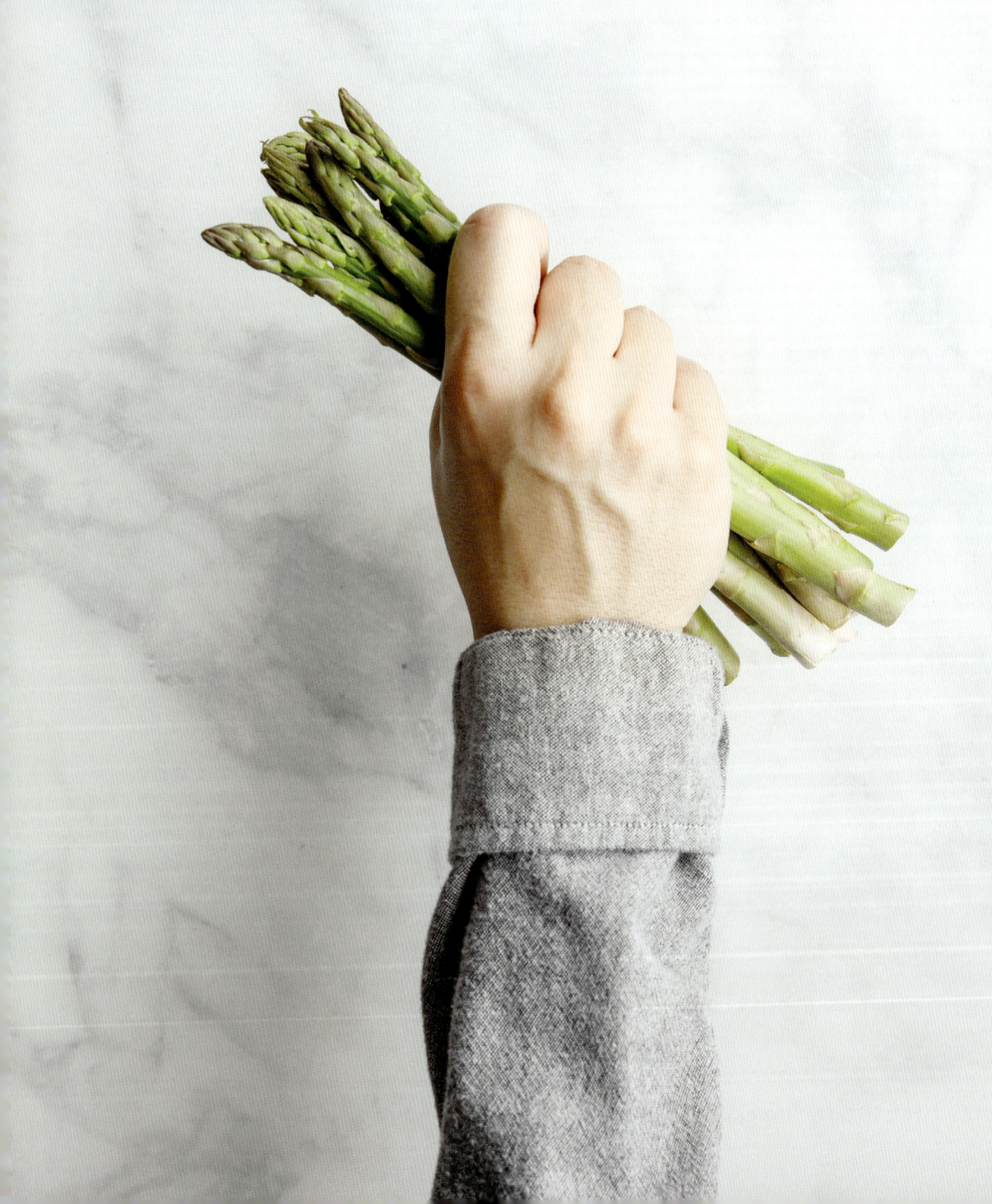

## recipes in this chapter...

**Herb-Infused Mock Mashed Potatoes, 183**

**Lemon Pepper Asparagus, 185**

**Spaghetti Squash, 186**

**Swiss Chard with Prosciutto and Pine Nuts, 187**

**Southern Collard Greens, 189**

**Creamed Kale, 190**

**Green Beans with Ham, 191**

**Instant Mock Mac and Cheese, 193**

**Sweet-and-Sour Red Cabbage, 194**

**Simply Steamed Broccoli, 195**

**Carbonara Brussels Sprouts, 197**

**Ratatouille, 199**

*Secret Message #8: We had to think long and hard about whether we should capitalize brussels sprouts as Brussels is a city, but capitalizing the vegetable has no consensus.*

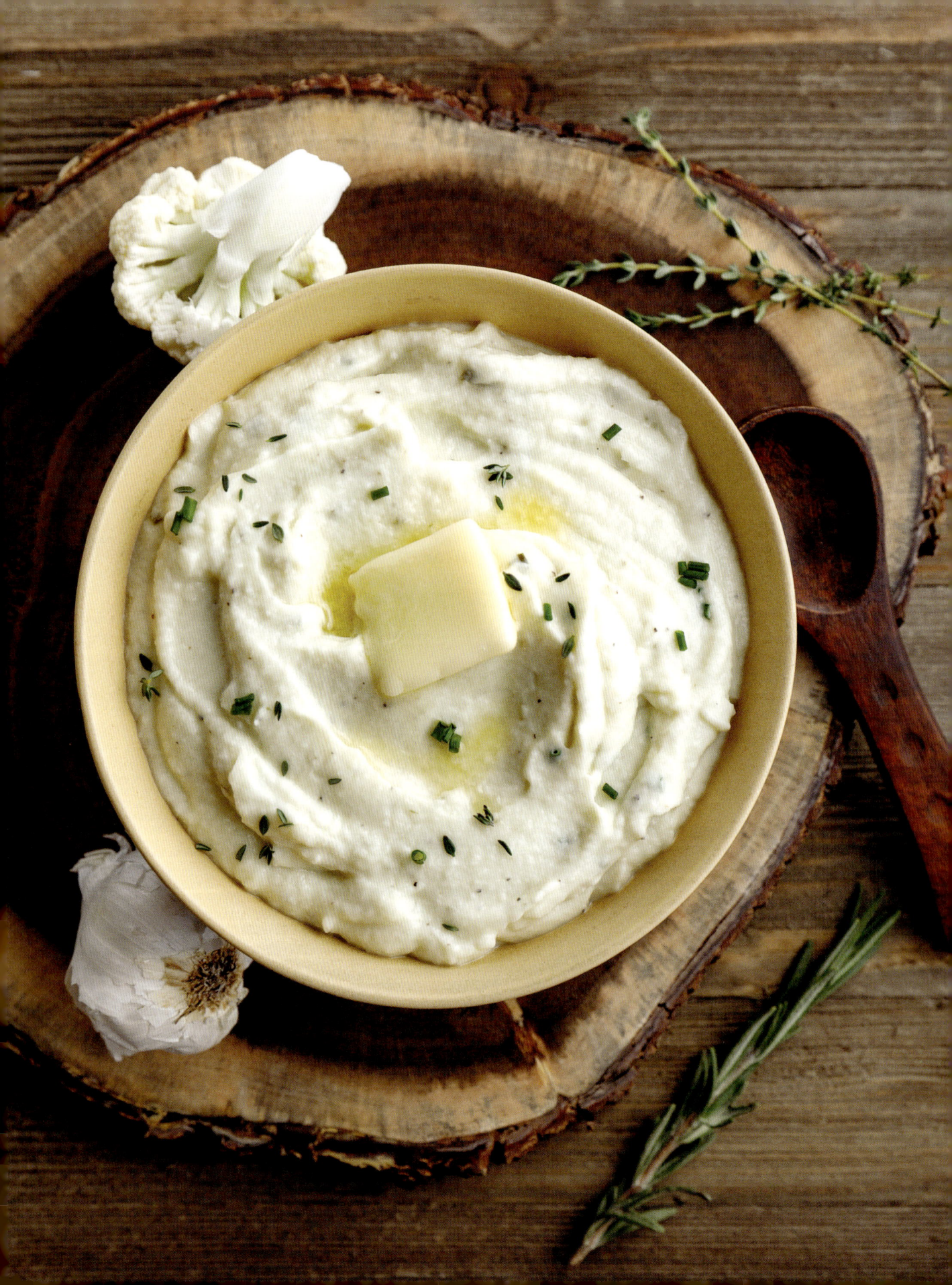

Prep Time: 10 min  |  High Pressure: 1 min  |  Quick Release  |  Serves: 4

# Herb-Infused Mock Mashed Potatoes

Thanks to the Instant Pot, making our classic cauliflower Mock Mashed Potatoes has never been quicker! In this variation on our low-carb staple, we've taken advantage of the closed environment of pressure cooking to infuse all the flavor of fresh herbs right into the cauliflower before mashing.

## Ingredients

1 cup chicken stock
2 cloves garlic
1 sprig fresh rosemary
2 sprigs fresh thyme
1 large head cauliflower, chopped
4 ounces herbed cream cheese
¼ cup grated Parmesan cheese
¼ teaspoon onion powder
Salt and pepper
Chopped chives, for garnish

## Special Equipment
Steam basket

1. Pour chicken stock into the Instant Pot and add garlic, rosemary, and thyme.
2. Insert steam basket over stock and herbs and add cauliflower to the basket.
3. Lock lid in place and seal pressure release vent. Set cooker to HIGH pressure for 1 minute.
4. Carefully open vent to quickly release the pressure.
5. Transfer cauliflower to a food processor and add cream cheese, Parmesan cheese, and onion powder. Discard chicken stock from the cooker.
6. Process cauliflower until smooth before seasoning with salt and pepper to taste. Serve topped with chopped chives, if desired.

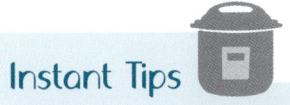

**Instant Tips**

Make classic Mock Mashed Potatoes by omitting the fresh rosemary and thyme and using regular cream cheese in place of the herbed cream cheese.

Calories: 175  |  Fat: 11.5g  |  Protein: 8.5g  |  Total Carbs: 10.5g  -  Fiber: 4g  =  Net Carbs: 6.5g

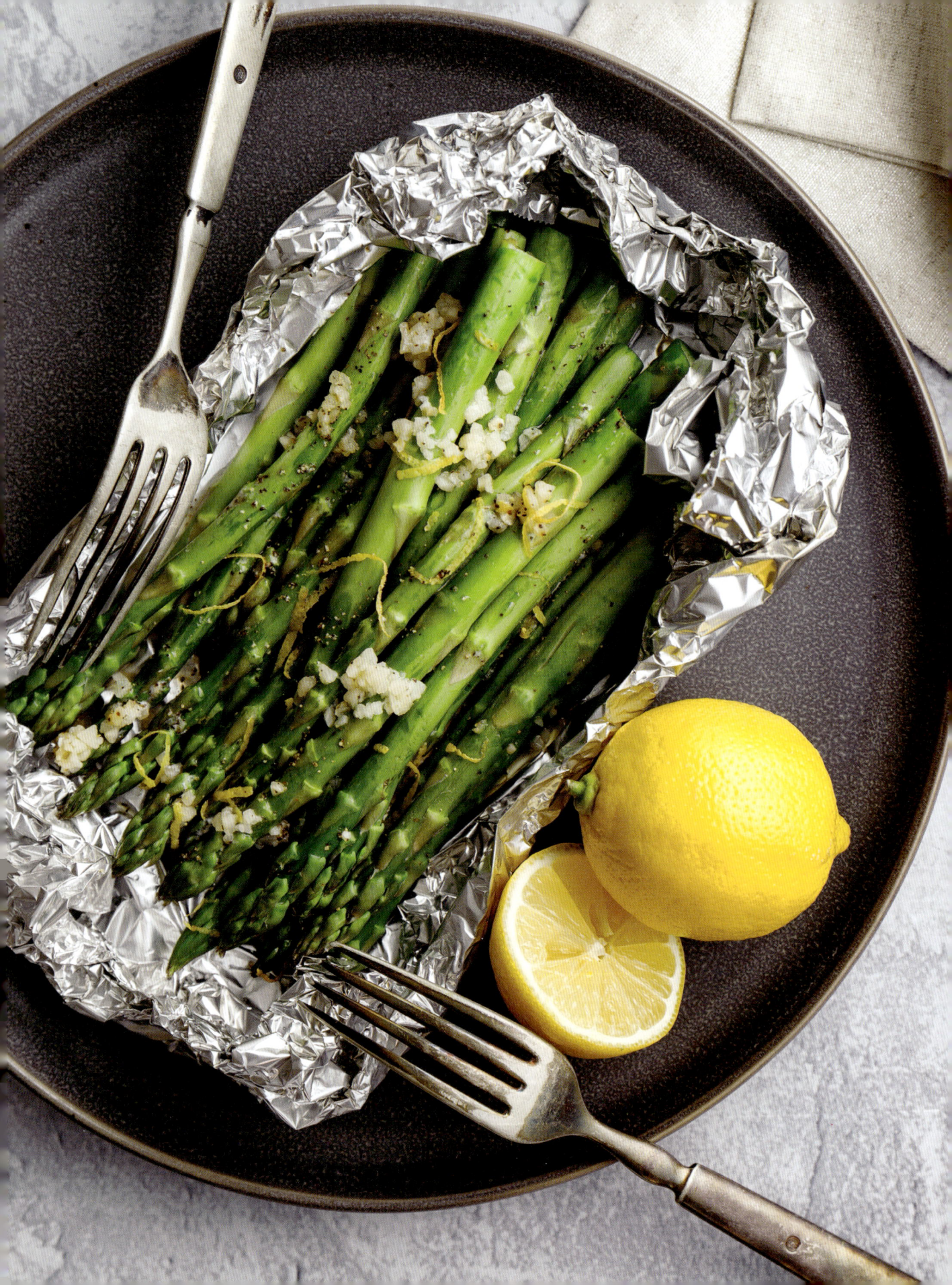

Prep Time: 10 min | High Pressure: 6 min | Quick Release | Serves: 4

# Lemon Pepper Asparagus

There is something oddly satisfying about cooking vegetables in a packet of aluminum foil, not just that it makes preparation (and cleanup!) less of a chore, but also the surprise of opening it up at the end of the cook time to find perfectly seasoned and tender-crisp asparagus spears that seemingly cooked themselves.

## Ingredients

1 bunch asparagus (up to 1 pound), stalks trimmed
2 tablespoons butter, chopped
1 teaspoon minced garlic
Zest of 1 small lemon
½ teaspoon cracked black pepper
¼ teaspoon salt

## Special Equipment

Steam rack

1. Pour 1 cup of water into the Instant Pot and insert steam rack.
2. Lay out a large square of aluminum foil and pile the asparagus up in the center.
3. Evenly disperse the butter, garlic, lemon zest, pepper, and salt over top the asparagus.
4. Fold the aluminum foil up to create a sealed packet. Place on steam rack in the cooker.
5. Lock lid in place and seal pressure release vent. Set cooker to HIGH pressure for 6 minutes. For pencil-thin asparagus, set cooker to HIGH for only 5 minutes.
6. Carefully open vent to quickly release the pressure.
7. Let cool 2 minutes before carefully opening the packet, as there will be steam inside.

**Instant Tips**

The cooking time in this recipe requires that you cook the asparagus in an aluminum foil packet, which takes a longer cook time but makes for stronger flavors.

Calories: 75 | Fat: 6g | Protein: 2.5g | Total Carbs: 4.5g - Fiber: 2.5g = Net Carbs: 2g

Prep Time: 10 min | High Pressure: 7 min | Quick Release | Serves: 4

# Spaghetti Squash

We used to bake our spaghetti squash in a water bath and it took AGES. With the Instant Pot, we can have this low-carb staple in just about 20 minutes.

## Ingredients

1 medium spaghetti squash

## Special Equipment

Steam rack

1. Pour 1 cup of water into the Instant Pot and insert steam rack.
2. Cut the spaghetti squash in half lengthwise.
3. Using a spoon, scrape out all seeds and the fibrous center around them.
4. Arrange the squash halves on the rack in any way that they will fit inside the cooker, even if they are tilted and slightly overlapped. It is best to keep them cut-side up.
5. Lock lid in place and seal pressure release vent. Set cooker to HIGH pressure for 7 minutes.
6. Carefully open vent to quickly release the pressure.
7. Let cool 5 minutes before using a fork to pull the strands of squash from the rind.

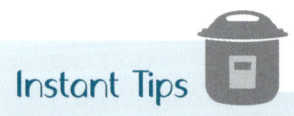

### Instant Tips

As a last resort, to fit the squash into the cooker, you can cut each half again to make quarters. You will just end up with smaller strands after cooking.

Calories: 30 | Fat: 0g | Protein: 0.5g | Total Carbs: 6.5g  -  Fiber: 1.5g  =  Net Carbs: 5g

Prep Time: 20 min | High Pressure: 3 min | Quick Release | Serves: 4

# Swiss Chard with Prosciutto and Pine Nuts

This deceptively simple side dish is elevated by toasted pine nuts and crispy prosciutto. It's the perfect pairing to a five-star meal at home.

## Ingredients

- 1 tablespoon olive oil
- 6 slices prosciutto, sliced into large strips
- 2 teaspoons minced garlic
- 1/2 cup chicken stock
- 1 tablespoon balsamic vinegar
- 2 teaspoons sugar substitute
- 1 large bunch Swiss chard, chopped
- Salt and pepper
- 1/4 cup toasted pine nuts (see tip)
- 2 tablespoons grated Parmesan cheese

1. Heat olive oil in the Instant Pot on the SAUTÉ setting.
2. Add prosciutto and cook until almost crispy before adding the garlic and sautéing just 1 minute more.
3. Stir in chicken stock, balsamic vinegar, and sugar substitute before topping with the chopped Swiss chard.
4. Lock lid in place and seal pressure release vent. Set cooker to HIGH pressure for 3 minutes.
5. Carefully open vent to quickly release the pressure.
6. Season with salt and pepper to taste before serving topped with the toasted pine nuts and grated Parmesan cheese.

### Instant Tips

You can now find toasted pine nuts for sale in some stores, but toasting your own is quite easy: Simply place in a sauté pan over medium heat and cook until golden brown and fragrant, about 5 minutes. For even toasting, be sure to shake the pan from time to time as the pine nuts cook.

Calories: 170 | Fat: 13g | Protein: 10.5g | Total Carbs: 5.5g - Fiber: 1.5g = Net Carbs: 4g

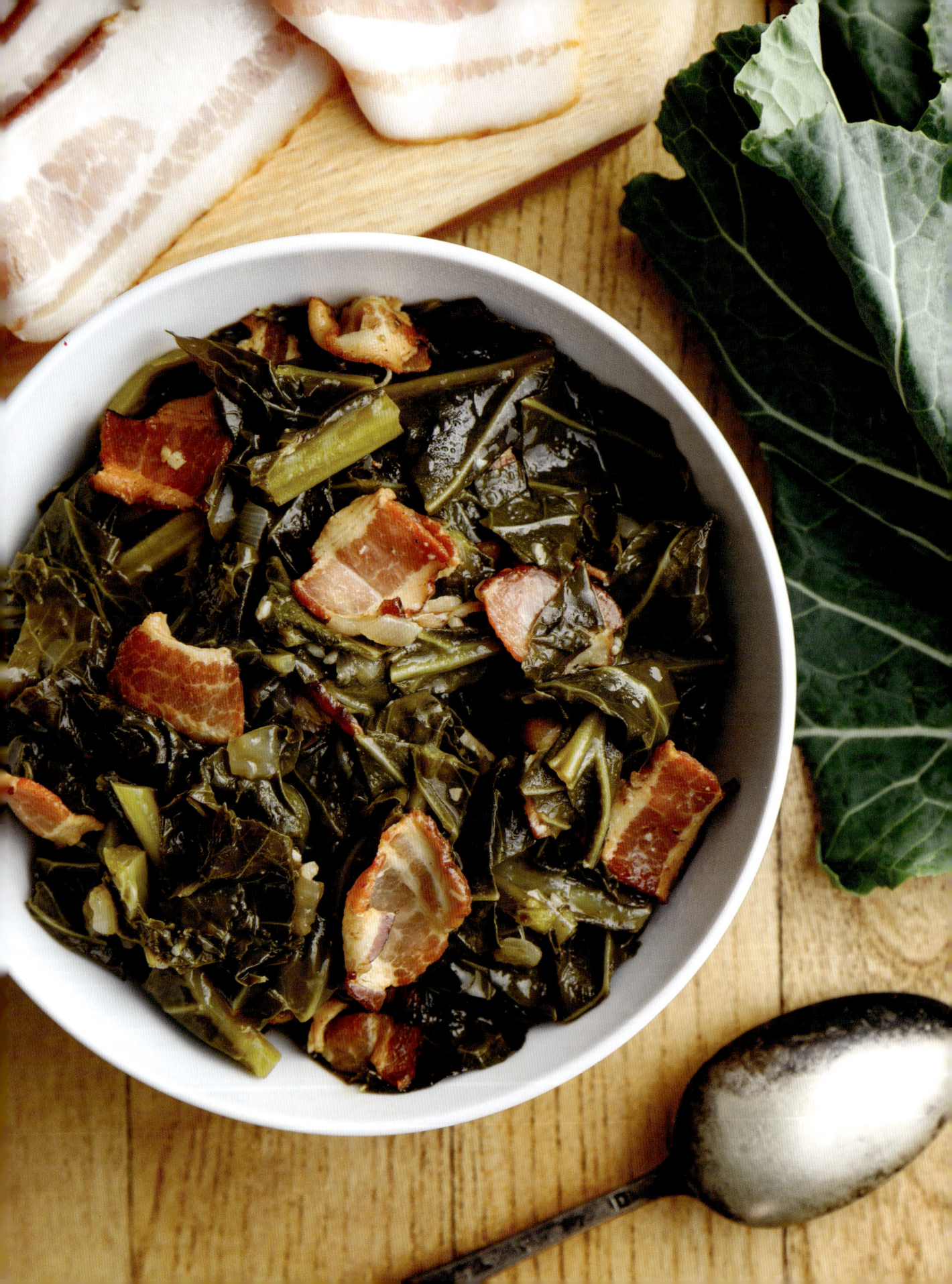

Prep Time: 10 min | High Pressure: 20 min | Natural Release: 5 min | Serves: 4

# Southern Collard Greens

The earthiness of the collard greens in this famous Southern side is offset by a bit of sweetness as well as a dash of Louisiana hot sauce. You'd be hard-pressed to find a better companion for anything with barbecue sauce... Or just plain anything at all!

## Ingredients

- 6 slices bacon, chopped
- 1/2 cup diced yellow onion
- 2 teaspoons minced garlic
- 1 cup chicken stock
- 1 tablespoon cider vinegar
- 1 tablespoon sugar substitute
- 2 teaspoons Louisiana hot sauce
- 1/2 teaspoon salt
- 1/2 teaspoon pepper
- 1 (16-ounce) bag chopped collard greens

1. Brown bacon in the Instant Pot on the SAUTÉ setting until bacon is almost crispy.
2. Add the onion and garlic and sauté 2 minutes or until onions begin to turn translucent.
3. Stir in chicken stock, cider vinegar, sugar substitute, hot sauce, salt, and pepper.
4. Add the collard greens and press down to ensure they are below the max-fill line.
5. Lock lid in place and seal pressure release vent. Set cooker to HIGH pressure for 20 minutes.
6. Let pressure release naturally for 5 minutes before opening vent to release any remaining pressure.
7. Adjust salt and pepper to taste before serving.

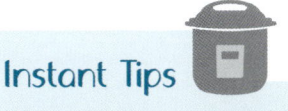

**Instant Tips**

You can also make this with a large bunch of fresh collard greens you chop yourself, but be sure to remove at least an inch of the stems, as they can be bitter and tough.

Calories: 115 | Fat: 4.5g | Protein: 7g | Total Carbs: 8g - Fiber: 3.5g = Net Carbs: 4.5g

Prep Time: 10 min | High Pressure: 3 min | Quick Release | Serves: 4–6

# Creamed Kale

Like creamed spinach but better, slightly sweet kale is smothered in a velvety cheese sauce in this simple side dish.

## Ingredients

1 tablespoon vegetable oil

½ cup diced red onion

2 teaspoons minced garlic

1 pound chopped kale

⅓ cup chicken stock

4 ounces cream cheese

¼ cup grated Parmesan cheese

Salt and pepper

1. Heat vegetable oil in the Instant Pot on the SAUTÉ setting.

2. Add the onion and garlic and sauté for 2 minutes or until fragrant. Stir in kale and chicken stock.

3. Lock lid in place and seal pressure release vent. Set cooker to HIGH pressure for 3 minutes.

4. Carefully open vent to quickly release the pressure.

5. Stir in cream cheese until fully melted into the sauce. To help with this process, you can set the cooker to SAUTÉ for about 1 minute, just long enough to get the cooker hot again after adding the cheese, but not long enough to burn it.

6. Stir in Parmesan cheese and season with salt and pepper to taste before serving.

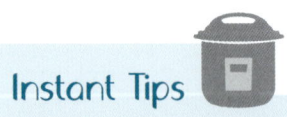

### Instant Tips

This can also be made with 10 to 12 ounces frozen chopped kale using only the SAUTÉ function on the Instant Pot until heated through, as you would not need to cook it under pressure.

Calories: 140 | Fat: 9g | Protein: 4.5g | Total Carbs: 10.5g - Fiber: 2g = Net Carbs: 8.5g

Prep Time: 10 min | High Pressure: 1 min | Quick Release | Serves: 4

# Green Beans with Ham

Besides the vivid color, perhaps the most beautiful thing about green beans is how wonderfully complementary they are. We wracked our brains trying to think of anything they wouldn't go with and came up with absolutely nothing! Serve this alongside chicken, pork, beef, or even... more ham!

## Ingredients

1 tablespoon butter

8 ounces diced ham

1/2 cup diced yellow onion

2 teaspoons minced garlic

1 pound green beans, trimmed

1/2 cup chicken stock

2 teaspoons sugar substitute

1/4 teaspoon onion powder

1/4 teaspoon salt

1/4 teaspoon pepper

1. Heat butter in the Instant Pot on the SAUTÉ setting.

2. Place ham, onion, and garlic in the cooker and sauté until onion is translucent and garlic is beginning to brown, about 5 minutes.

3. For the best texture, transfer ham and onion to a bowl and set aside until after pressure cooking the beans.

4. Add green beans, chicken stock, sugar substitute, onion powder, salt, and pepper to the cooker and toss to combine.

5. Lock lid in place and seal pressure release vent. Set cooker to HIGH pressure for 1 minute.

6. Carefully open vent to quickly release the pressure.

7. Add the ham and onion back into the cooker and toss with the beans to heat everything back through. Serve immediately.

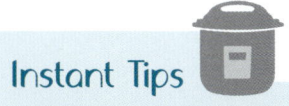

### Instant Tips

We like to cut the green beans into 1 1/2-inch lengths for this recipe, as it makes it easier to get both the beans and ham on your fork at the same time.

Calories: 125 | Fat: 4g | Protein: 12.5g | Total Carbs: 11g - Fiber: 4g = Net Carbs: 7g

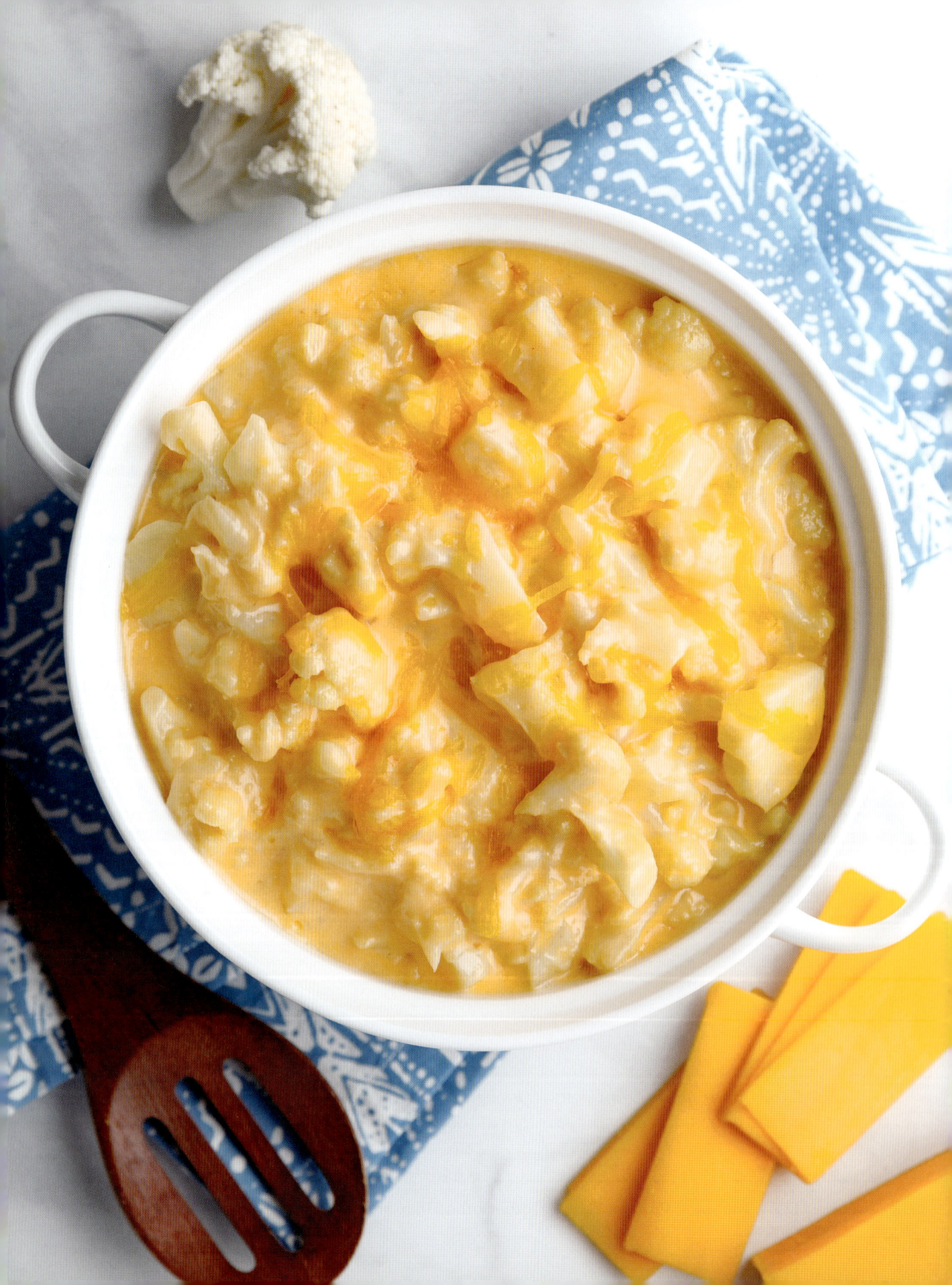

Prep Time: 10 min | High Pressure: 0 min | Quick Release | Serves: 4

# Instant Mock Mac and Cheese

Mock Mac and Cheese was one of the first recipes we wrote when we started the low-carb lifestyle. Nearly two decades later, we're still thinking up ways to make it even better—adding a touch of ground mustard to the cheese sauce for an extra layer of flavor—and now, under pressure, it's our fastest Mock Mac and Cheese yet.

## Ingredients

²/₃ cup chicken stock

1 head cauliflower, chopped into ³/₄-inch pieces

½ cup heavy cream

1 ½ cups shredded sharp Cheddar cheese

2 ounces cream cheese

¼ teaspoon ground mustard

¼ teaspoon salt

¼ teaspoon pepper

## Special Equipment

Steam basket

1. Pour chicken stock into the Instant Pot and place steam basket in cooker. Add cauliflower to the steam basket.

2. Lock lid in place and seal pressure release vent. Set cooker to HIGH pressure for 0 minutes.

3. Carefully open vent to quickly release the pressure.

4. Drain ³/₄ of the liquid from the cooker before transferring cauliflower from the steam basket to the inner pot.

5. Set cooker to SAUTÉ and stir in heavy cream, bringing up to a simmer. Turn off cooker.

6. Add all remaining ingredients and stir until cheese has melted and all is combined. Serve immediately.

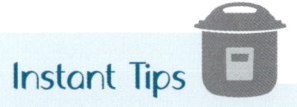

### Instant Tips

We've also made this without the steam basket, and it has turned out almost entirely the same, but the basket does make draining the liquid an easier process.

Calories: 355 | Fat: 31.5g | Protein: 13g | Total Carbs: 9.5g - Fiber: 3.5g = Net Carbs: 6g

Prep Time: 10 min | High Pressure: 5 min | Quick Release | Serves: 6

# Sweet-and-Sour Red Cabbage

This quick-pickled cabbage is fantastic when served warm as a side dish or chilled as a condiment for pork or sausages.

## Ingredients

1 small head red cabbage, shredded

¼ cup red wine vinegar

2 ½ tablespoons sugar substitute

2 tablespoons water

¼ teaspoon salt

2 tablespoons butter

1. Add cabbage, vinegar, sugar substitute, water, and salt to the Instant Pot and toss to coat cabbage.
2. Lock lid in place and seal pressure release vent. Set cooker to HIGH pressure for 5 minutes.
3. Carefully open vent to quickly release the pressure.
4. Stir in butter before serving.

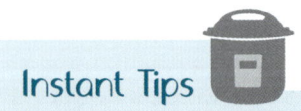

**Instant Tips**

This can also be made with a bag of shredded coleslaw mix; however, the green cabbage in the mix will not have as nice of a presentation as the red cabbage you'd shred yourself.

Calories: 65 | Fat: 4g | Protein: 1.5g | Total Carbs: 7g - Fiber: 2.5g = Net Carbs: 4.5g

Prep Time: 5 min | High Pressure: 1 min | Quick Release | Serves: 4

# Simply Steamed Broccoli

Sometimes, the best side dish is the simplest side dish! That said, broccoli is probably the easiest vegetable to overcook in a pressure cooker, which is why we follow these cook times. Our favorite way to season it after cooking? We sprinkle it with grated Parmesan cheese and black pepper while it is still hot.

## Ingredients

1 bunch broccoli

Vegetable or chicken stock

Aromatics (lemon wedges, garlic cloves, fresh herbs)

Salt and pepper

## Special Equipment

Steam basket

1. Pour 1 cup of water into the Instant Pot and insert steam basket. For more flavor, use vegetable or chicken stock in place of the water.

2. For even more flavor, you can add aromatics such as whole lemon wedges, garlic cloves, or fresh herbs to the cooking liquid.

3. Cut the large stalk from the broccoli and discard (see tip). Cut the rest of the broccoli into large florets. Transfer florets to the steam basket.

4. Lock lid in place and seal pressure release vent. For crisp and fresh broccoli: Set cooker to HIGH pressure for 1 minute. For tender broccoli: Set cooker to HIGH pressure for 2 minutes.

5. Carefully open vent to quickly release the pressure. Be sure to do this as soon as the time has elapsed or the broccoli will overcook!

6. To retain texture, steam basket should be removed from the cooker as soon as possible; otherwise, the residual heat will continue steaming it.

7. Season with salt and pepper to taste while the broccoli is still steaming hot.

### Instant Tips

The stem can be chopped up and added to soups as an alternative to chopped potatoes. If cooked until soft, you can blend the stem to thicken soups without the carbs of other thickeners.

---

Calories: 50 | Fat: 0.5g | Protein: 4g | Total Carbs: 10g - Fiber: 4g = Net Carbs: 6g

Instant Low Carb

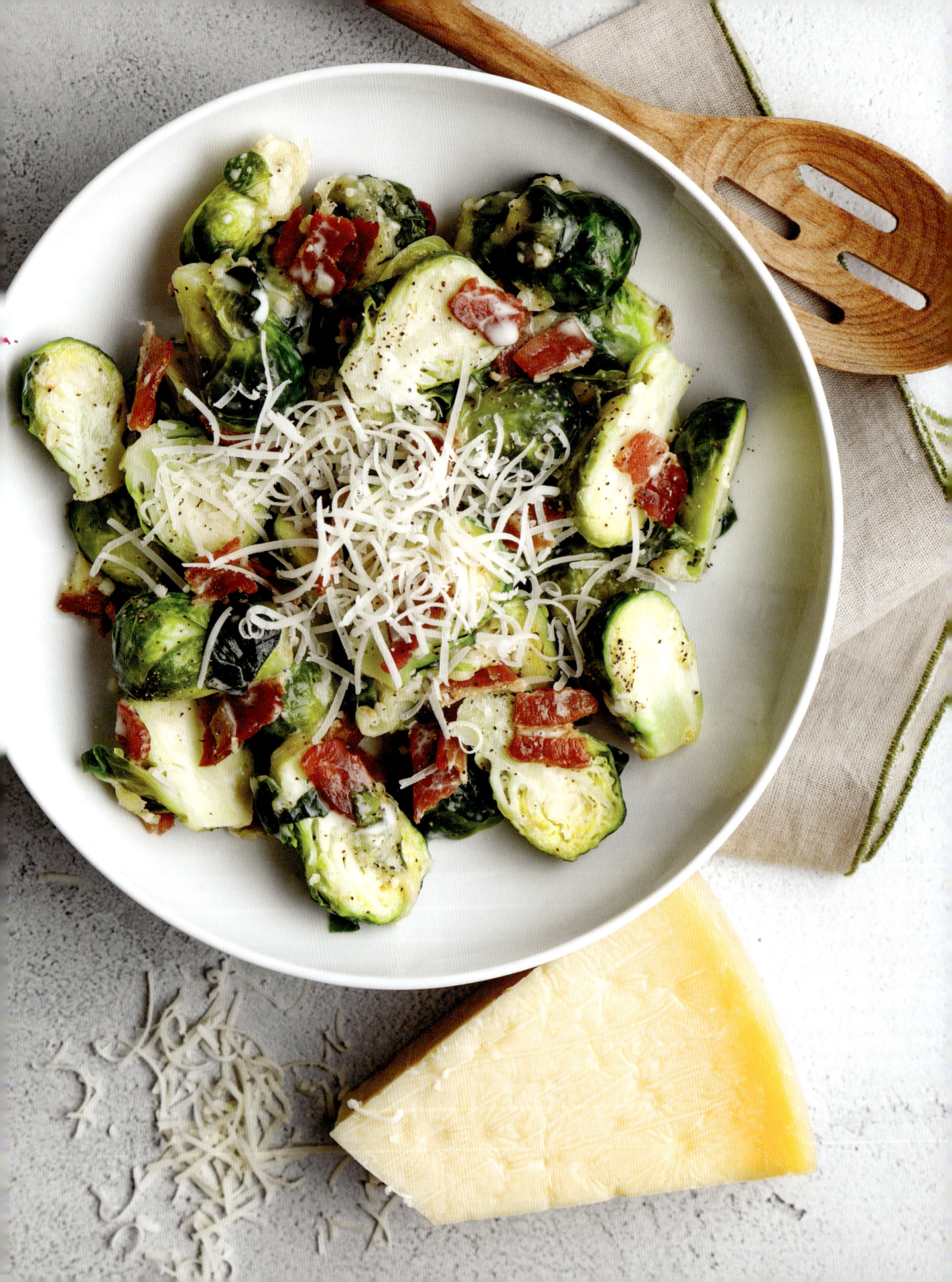

Prep Time: 10 min  |  High Pressure: 1 min  |  Quick Release  |  Serves: 4

# Carbonara Brussels Sprouts

These brussels sprouts with crispy bacon in a Parmesan cream sauce (think Alfredo Sauce) are a quick side that really spruces up the humble sprout.

## Ingredients

6 slices bacon, chopped
1 tablespoon minced garlic
½ cup chicken stock
1 pound brussels sprouts, halved
⅓ cup heavy cream
½ cup grated Parmesan cheese
Salt and pepper

## Special Equipment

Steam basket

1. Heat bacon in the Instant Pot set to SAUTÉ, cooking until browned and crispy. Stir in garlic and sauté for 1 additional minute.

2. Remove bacon from cooker and discard bacon grease.

3. Pour chicken stock into the Instant Pot and place steam basket in cooker. Add brussels sprouts to the steam basket.

4. Lock lid in place and seal pressure release vent. Set cooker to HIGH pressure for 1 minute.

5. Carefully open vent to quickly release the pressure.

6. Drain ¾ of the liquid from the cooker before transferring brussels sprouts from the steam basket to the inner pot.

7. Set cooker to SAUTÉ and stir in heavy cream, bringing up to a simmer. Let simmer 2 minutes to slightly thicken.

8. Turn off cooker and stir in Parmesan cheese and cooked bacon. Season with salt and pepper to taste before serving.

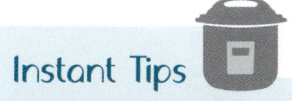

> **Instant Tips**
>
> For a dish that is closer to a true carbonara from Italy, use ¾ cup of diced pancetta in place of the chopped bacon.

Calories: 225  |  Fat: 17g  |  Protein: 13g  |  Total Carbs: 10g  -  Fiber: 4g  =  Net Carbs: 6g

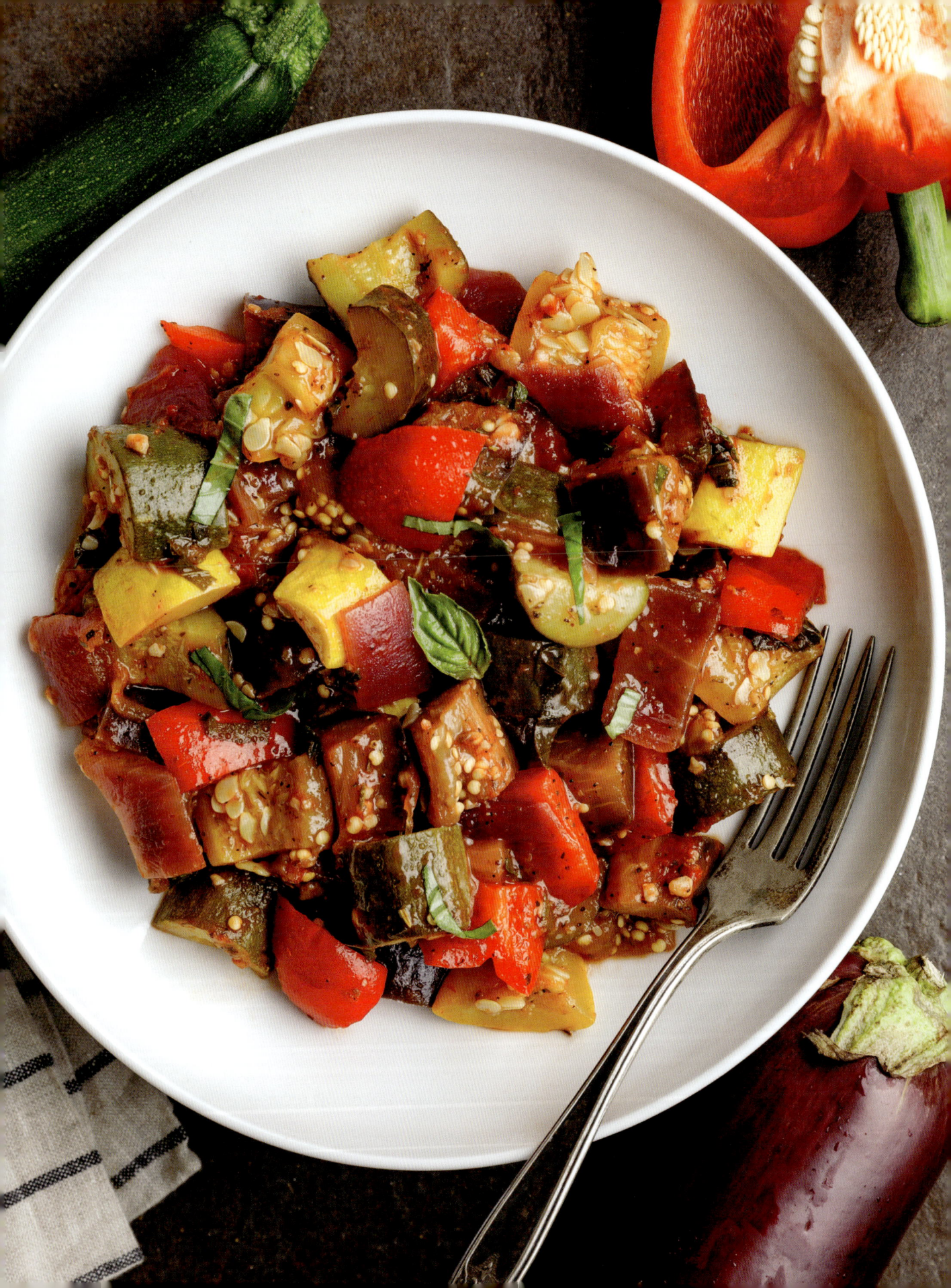

Prep Time: 20 min | High Pressure: 3 min | Quick Release | Serves: 6

# Ratatouille

Since there are plenty of natural carbs in the fresh vegetables used in this stew, we opted to omit the higher-carb diced or fresh tomatoes and only added a bit of tomato paste, just enough for the broth to retain its characteristic tomato flavor while also allowing the other ingredients to shine.

## Ingredients

2 tablespoons olive oil

1/2 small red onion, chopped

1/2 red bell pepper, chopped

1 tablespoon minced garlic

3 cups chopped yellow squash

3 cups chopped eggplant

2 cups chopped zucchini

2/3 cup vegetable stock

1/4 cup chopped fresh basil, divided

1 tablespoon balsamic vinegar

2 teaspoons Italian seasoning

3/4 teaspoon salt

1/2 teaspoon pepper

2 tablespoons tomato paste

1. Heat olive oil in the Instant Pot on the SAUTÉ setting.

2. Add onion, bell pepper, and garlic and sauté for 3 minutes or until onions begin to turn translucent.

3. Fold in all remaining ingredients except tomato paste and 1/2 of the fresh basil.

4. Lock lid in place and seal pressure release vent. Set cooker to HIGH pressure for 3 minutes.

5. Carefully open vent to quickly release the pressure.

6. Drain 1/2 of the liquid from the cooker before stirring in tomato paste and the remaining 1/2 of fresh basil.

### Instant Tips

For the most even cooking, be sure to chop all of your vegetables to a similar size and shape. Larger pieces will hold their shape better, and smaller pieces will result in a final dish that is softer and more of a stew.

Calories: 80 | Fat: 5g | Protein: 2g | Total Carbs: 8.5g - Fiber: 3g = Net Carbs: 5.5g

*Chapter 9*

# Desserts

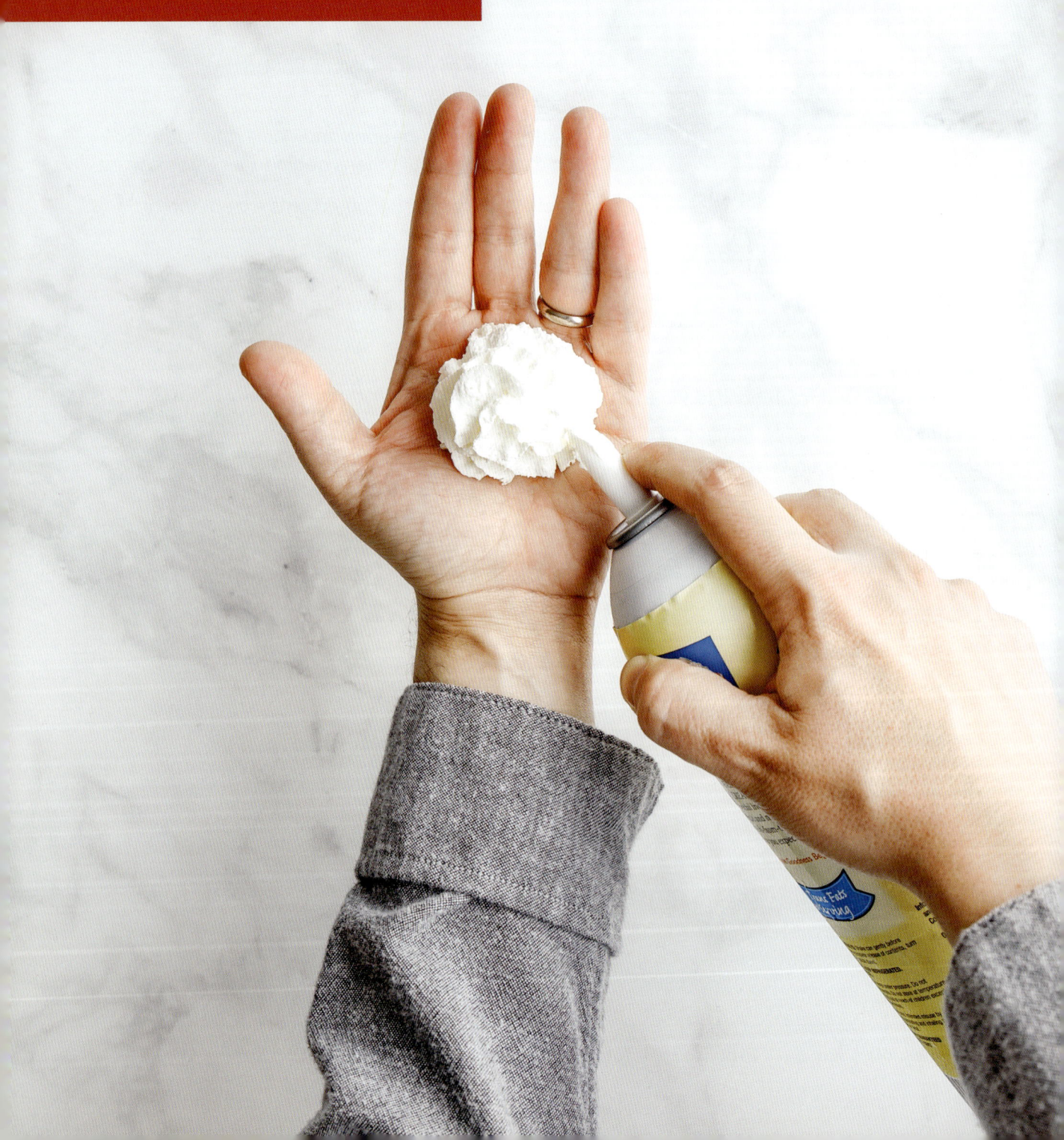

## recipes in this chapter...

**Instant Cheesecake**, 203
**Peanut Pots de Crème**, 205
**Cappuccino Flan**, 207
**Fudge Brownie Soufflé Cups**, 209
**Orange and Cream Cheesecake Bites**, 210
**Mixed Berry Sauce**, 211
**Angel Bar Cake**, 213
**Mexican Hot Chocolate**, 215
**Raspberry Cheesecake Bites**, 217
**Key Lime Custard Cups**, 219

Secret Message #9: Everyone keeps seeing funny faces in the swirls of hot chocolate on page 214. The one on the right looks like a pug.

*Desserts*

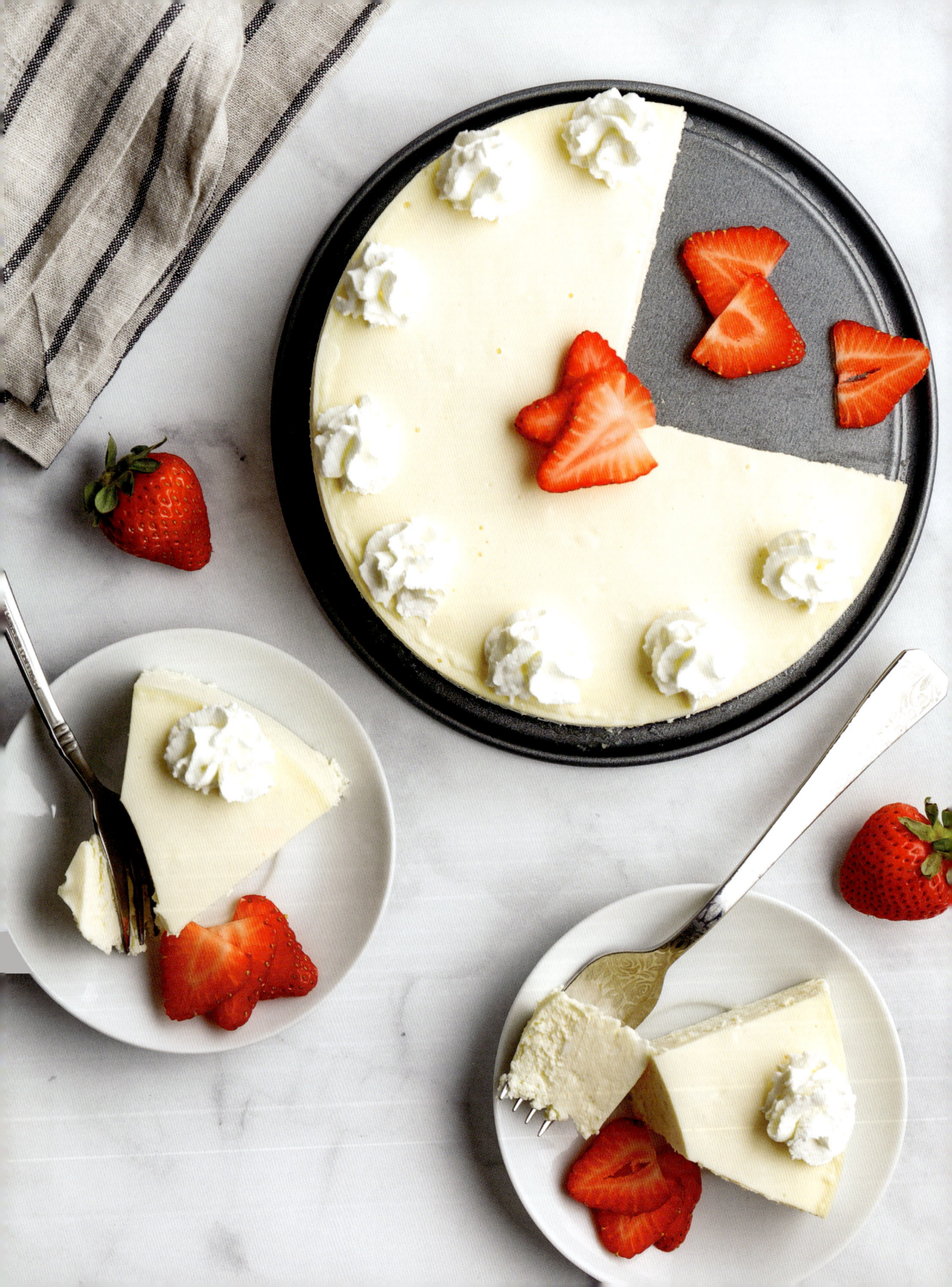

Prep Time: 10 min | High Pressure: 25 min | Natural Release: 15 min | Serves: 8

# Instant Cheesecake

Cheesecakes have always been our specialty and just so happen to be the top dessert to prepare in a pressure cooker. Unlike oven preparations, there's no risk of the cake drying out or cracking—just an evenly cooked cake every time. The batter in this particular recipe has been tweaked from our classic recipes to make it as simple and foolproof as possible.

## Ingredients

Nonstick cooking spray
1 pound cream cheese
2 large eggs
1 large egg yolk
¼ cup heavy cream
⅔ cup sugar substitute
1 teaspoon vanilla extract

## Special Equipment

7-inch springform pan
Steam rack

1. For best results, start with cream cheese, eggs, and heavy cream at room temperature.

2. Pour 1 cup of water into the Instant Pot. Spray a 7-inch springform pan with nonstick cooking spray.

3. In an electric mixer, beat all remaining ingredients until smooth and combined.

4. Pour the batter into the prepared cake pan and tap against the counter to remove any air bubbles. Tightly wrap the bottom and top of the pan to ensure it is watertight before placing on steam rack. Carefully lower into the water bath in the Instant Pot.

5. Lock lid in place and seal pressure release vent. Set cooker to HIGH pressure for 25 minutes.

6. Let pressure release naturally for 15 minutes before opening vent to release any remaining pressure.

7. Cool on counter for at least 30 minutes, then chill at least 4 hours before slicing to serve.

### Instant Tips

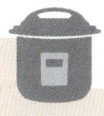

Some water usually condensates on the top of the cheesecake during the cooking process. We lightly pat the top of the cake with a paper towel after cooling on the counter, but before refrigerating, just to ensure the water doesn't seep back into the cake.

Calories: 260 | Fat: 24.5g | Protein: 6g | Total Carbs: 4g - Fiber: 0g = Net Carbs: 4g

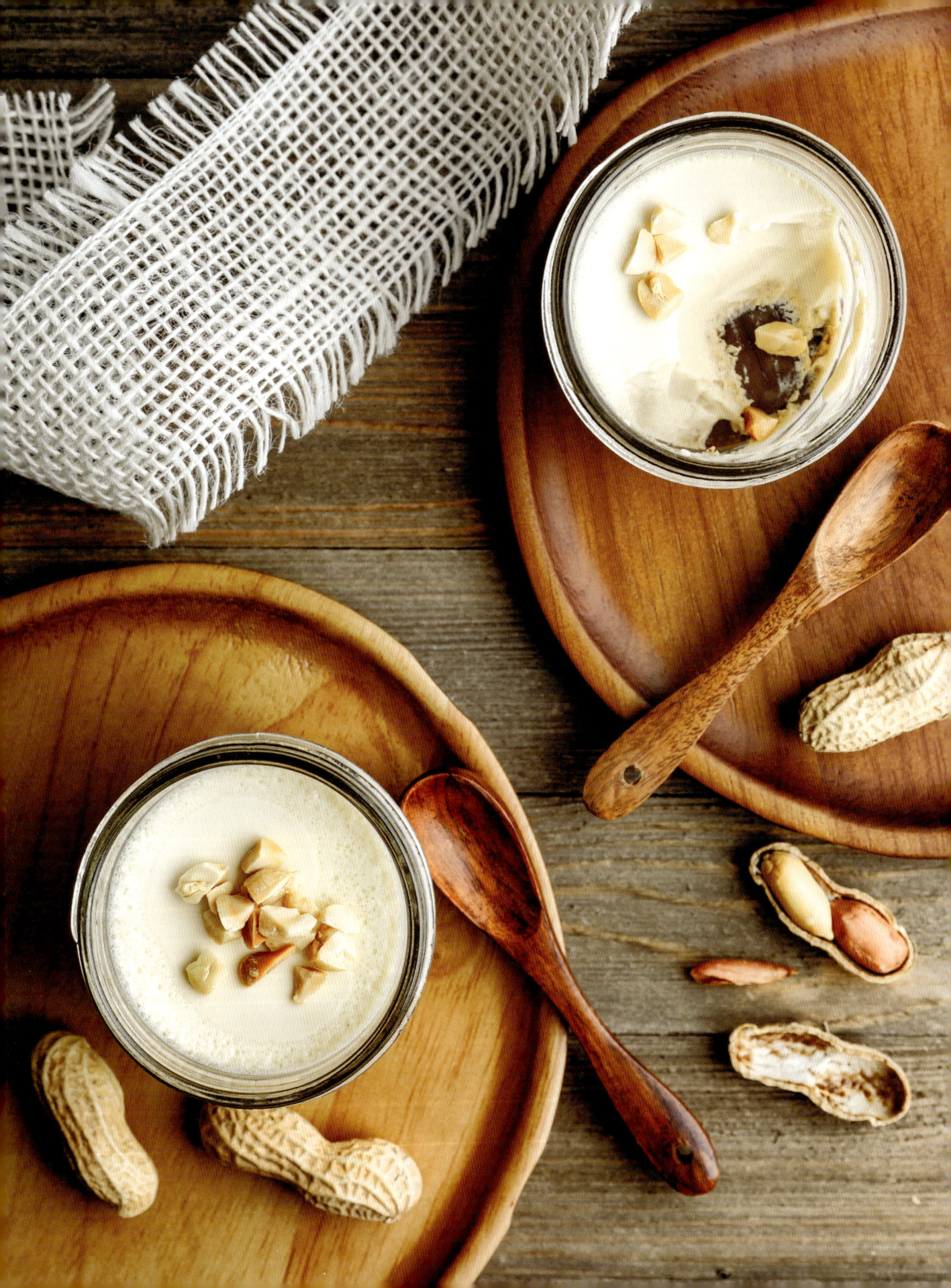

**Prep Time:** 15 min | **High Pressure:** 7 min | **Natural Release:** 5 min | **Serves:** 4

# Peanut Pots de Crème

While it may seem too simple, this peanut-flavored custard is actually our favorite dessert in this section. We like to make these in small heatproof jars (suitable for canning), but they can also be made in ramekins. Some peanut powder will naturally settle on the bottom of the jar and rehydrate into a thin layer of peanut butter you can spoon out. Serve topped with chopped peanuts, sugar-free whipped cream, or both.

## Ingredients

¾ cup heavy cream

½ cup unsweetened almond milk

⅓ cup sugar substitute

¼ teaspoon vanilla extract

3 large egg yolks

¼ cup powdered peanut butter (see tip)

## Special Equipment

4 ramekins

Steam rack

1. Pour 1 cup of water into the Instant Pot.
2. In a saucepot on the stove set to medium heat, whisk together heavy cream, almond milk, sugar substitute, and vanilla extract. Whisking occasionally, bring up to a low simmer and immediately remove from heat.
3. Meanwhile, in a mixing bowl, whisk the egg yolks together.
4. While whisking constantly, slowly pour the hot cream into the egg yolk mixture until combined.
5. Whisk the powdered peanut butter into the cream and egg mixture. For the best presentation, use a spoon to skim off any foam from the top of the mixture.
6. Divide the mixture evenly between 4 ramekins and cover with aluminum foil. Place on steam rack and lower into the water bath in the cooker.
7. Lock lid in place and seal pressure release vent. Set cooker to HIGH pressure for 7 minutes.
8. Let pressure release naturally for 5 minutes before opening vent to let out remaining pressure.
9. Let cool on counter for at least 30 minutes before refrigerating at least 3 hours. Serve chilled.

### Instant Tips

Peanut butter powder is most often sold near the regular peanut butter but can sometimes be found in the health food aisle. We look for a brand without any added sugar.

**Calories:** 235 | **Fat:** 21.5g | **Protein:** 5.5g | **Total Carbs:** 6g  -  **Fiber:** 1g  =  **Net Carbs:** 5g

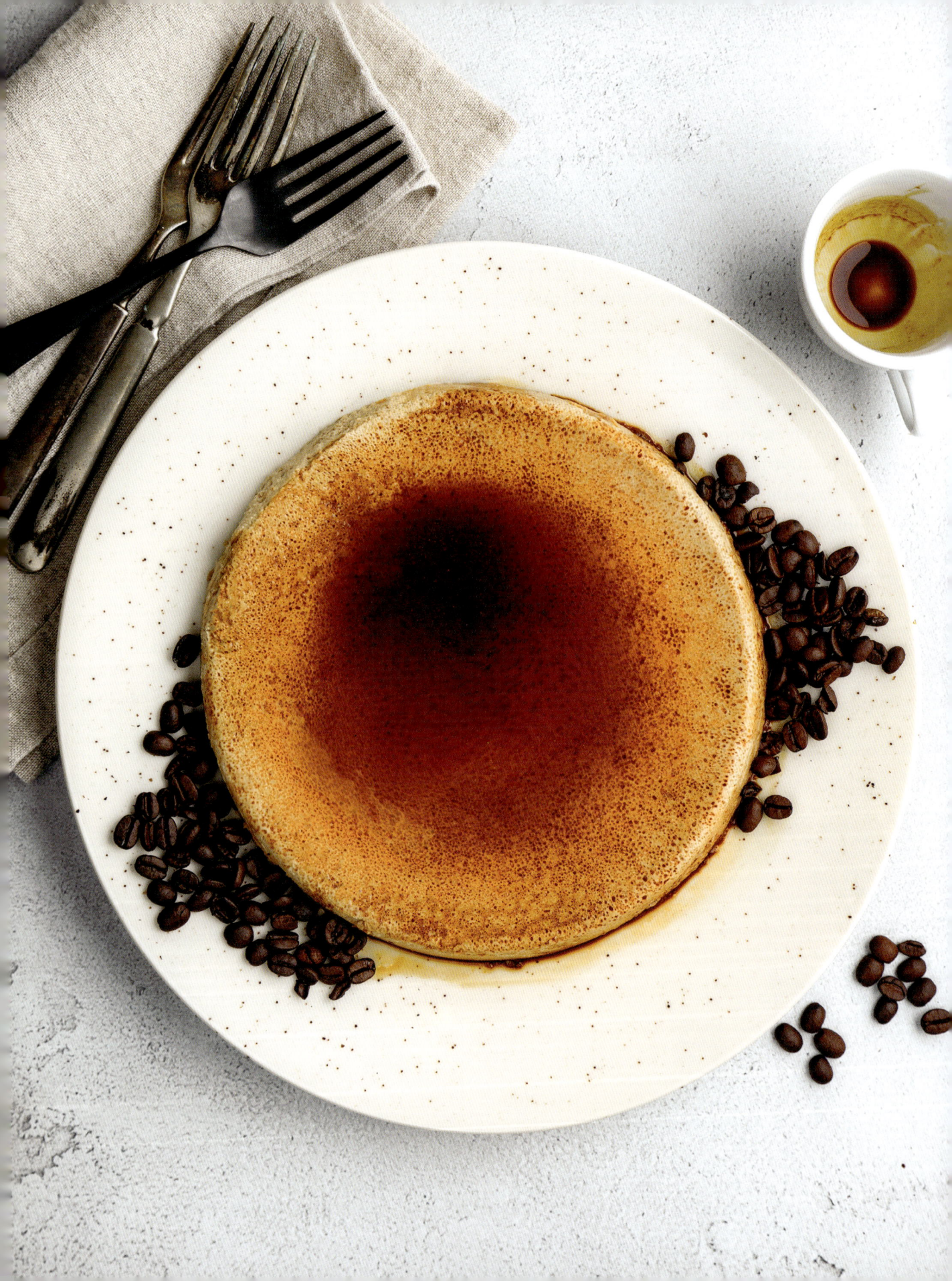

Prep Time: 5 min | High Pressure: 10 min | Natural Release: 12 min | Serves: 6

# Cappuccino Flan

Flan is the perfect Instant Pot dessert, as it is traditionally made by steaming in a water bath and doesn't do well when introduced to the dry heat of an oven. In our recipe, we've added instant coffee granules to the custard for that cappuccino flavor without adding additional liquid. The coffee syrup topping is optional but highly recommended. Without the coffee syrup, this is also delicious topped with a sprinkling of sugar substitute and ground cinnamon.

## Ingredients

Nonstick cooking spray
1 cup heavy cream
3 large eggs
Rounded 1/3 cup sugar substitute
1 tablespoon instant coffee granules
1/4 teaspoon vanilla extract

### Coffee Syrup

1 cup strong brewed coffee or 1/2 cup espresso
2 tablespoons sugar substitute

### Special Equipment

7-inch cake pan or springform pan
Steam rack

1. Pour 1 cup of water into the Instant Pot. Spray a 7-inch metal cake pan with nonstick cooking spray.

2. In a mixing bowl, whisk together heavy cream, eggs, sugar substitute, coffee granules, and vanilla extract until smooth and combined.

3. Pour the egg mixture into the prepared cake pan, cover tightly with aluminum foil, and place on a steam rack. Carefully lower into the water bath in the Instant Pot.

4. Lock lid in place and seal pressure release vent. Set cooker to HIGH pressure for 10 minutes.

5. Let pressure release naturally for 12 minutes before opening vent to release any remaining pressure.

6. Cool on counter for 30 minutes, then chill at least 4 hours before serving. To serve, run a knife along the outer edges to release flan from the pan, then invert onto a serving plate.

**Coffee Syrup:** Create a coffee syrup to pour over top the flan by adding the coffee and sugar substitute to a small saucepan over medium-high heat. Bring up to a boil and let reduce for about 10 minutes, until only 2 tablespoons of liquid remains. Chill alongside flan until ready to serve.

### Instant Tips

I've found that 1/2 cup of sugar substitute in the flan is too much and 1/3 cup is too little, so rounding the 1/3 cup measuring cup or using 1/3 cup plus 2 tablespoons is perfect.

Calories: 185 | Fat: 17.5g | Protein: 4g | Total Carbs: 3g - Fiber: 0g = Net Carbs: 3g

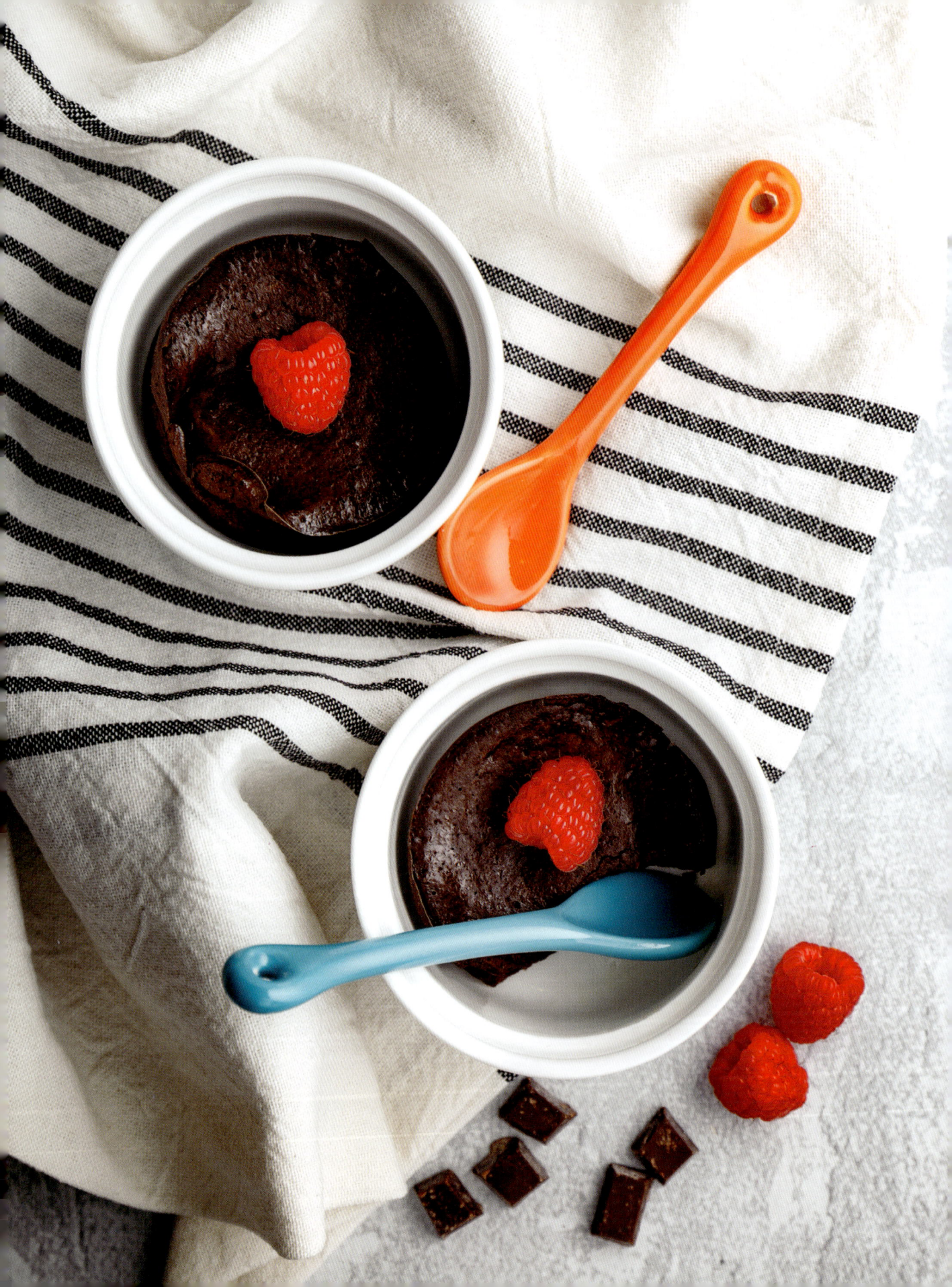

**Prep Time: 10 min | High Pressure: 6 min | Quick Release | Serves: 3**

# Fudge Brownie Soufflé Cups

These rich chocolate cups rise right in the Instant Pot without the hassles of baking traditional soufflés. It's a great big blast of chocolate that makes the perfect low-carb stand-in for brownies or fudge.

## Ingredients

Nonstick cooking spray

4 tablespoons unsalted butter, melted

¼ cup sugar substitute

1 large egg

1 large egg white

2 tablespoons unsweetened cocoa powder

¼ teaspoon vanilla extract

¼ teaspoon baking powder

## Special Equipment

3 ramekins

Steam rack

1. Pour 1 cup of water into the Instant Pot. Spray 3 ramekins with nonstick cooking spray.
2. In a mixing bowl, whisk together all remaining ingredients to create a batter.
3. Spoon an equal amount of the batter into each prepared ramekin. Tap each ramekin on the counter to even out the top of the batter.
4. Cover each ramekin tightly with aluminum foil, then arrange all 3 on the steam rack. Carefully lower into the water bath in the Instant Pot.
5. Lock lid in place and seal pressure release vent. Set cooker to HIGH pressure for 6 minutes.
6. Carefully open vent to quickly release the pressure. Serve warm, right out of the ramekins.

### Instant Tips

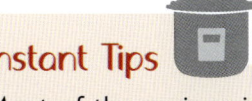

Most of the recipes in this book work fine whether they are made with salted or unsalted butter but we've found that this specific recipe can be a bit too salty when made with salted butter.

**Calories: 185 | Fat: 17.5g | Protein: 4g | Total Carbs: 4.5g - Fiber: 1g = Net Carbs: 3.5g**

Prep Time: 10 min | High Pressure: 12 min | Natural Release: 15 min | Serves: 7

# Orange and Cream Cheesecake Bites

These Creamsicle-inspired cheesecake bites are made with fresh orange zest for a full flavor that is all natural.

## Ingredients

Nonstick cooking spray
8 ounces cream cheese
1/3 cup sugar substitute
1/4 cup heavy cream
1 large egg
1 large egg yolk
Zest of 1 small orange
1/2 teaspoon vanilla extract

## Special Equipment

Egg bites mold
Steam rack

1. For best results, start with all ingredients at room temperature.
2. Pour 1 cup of water into the Instant Pot. Spray egg bites mold with nonstick cooking spray.
3. Place all remaining ingredients in a food processor and process just until smooth.
4. Evenly pour the batter into each cup of the egg bites mold. Tap the mold against the counter to remove any air bubbles before wrapping with aluminum foil.
5. Place egg bites mold on steam rack and lower into the water bath in the cooker.
6. Lock lid in place and seal pressure release vent. Set cooker to HIGH pressure for 12 minutes.
7. Let pressure release naturally for 15 minutes before opening vent to release any remaining pressure.
8. Cool on counter for at least 30 minutes, then chill at least 2 hours before popping out of mold to serve.

### Instant Tips

This same method can be done with zest from a large lemon, 2 limes, or 1/2 grapefruit to make cheesecake bites in other citrus flavors.

Calories: 165 | Fat: 15.5g | Protein: 4g | Total Carbs: 2.5g - Fiber: 0g = Net Carbs: 2.5g

**Prep Time: 5 min** | **High Pressure: 3 min** | **Natural Release: 2 min** | **Serves: 8**

# Mixed Berry Sauce

This berry sauce, made with an inexpensive bag of frozen mixed berries, is a perfect topping for other low-carb desserts. It's especially great when drizzled over our Instant Cheesecake (page: 203) or Angel Bar Cake (page: 213).

## Ingredients

1 (12-ounce) package frozen mixed berries

½ cup sugar substitute

¼ cup water

¼ teaspoon vanilla extract

1. Add all ingredients to the Instant Pot and stir to combine.
2. Lock lid in place and seal pressure release vent. Set cooker to HIGH pressure for 3 minutes.
3. Let pressure release naturally for 2 minutes before carefully opening the vent to let out remaining pressure.
4. Use a heavy spoon or potato masher to mash any large berries into the sauce.
5. For a slightly thicker texture, set cooker to SAUTÉ and bring up to a simmer. Let sauce reduce for 3 minutes.
6. Serve warm or chilled. Sauce will thicken further when chilled.

### Instant Tips

We tried making this with fresh berries but it was expensive and actually had a less concentrated flavor.

**Calories: 30** | **Fat: 0g** | **Protein: 0g** | **Total Carbs: 6.5g** - **Fiber: 1.5g** = **Net Carbs: 5g**

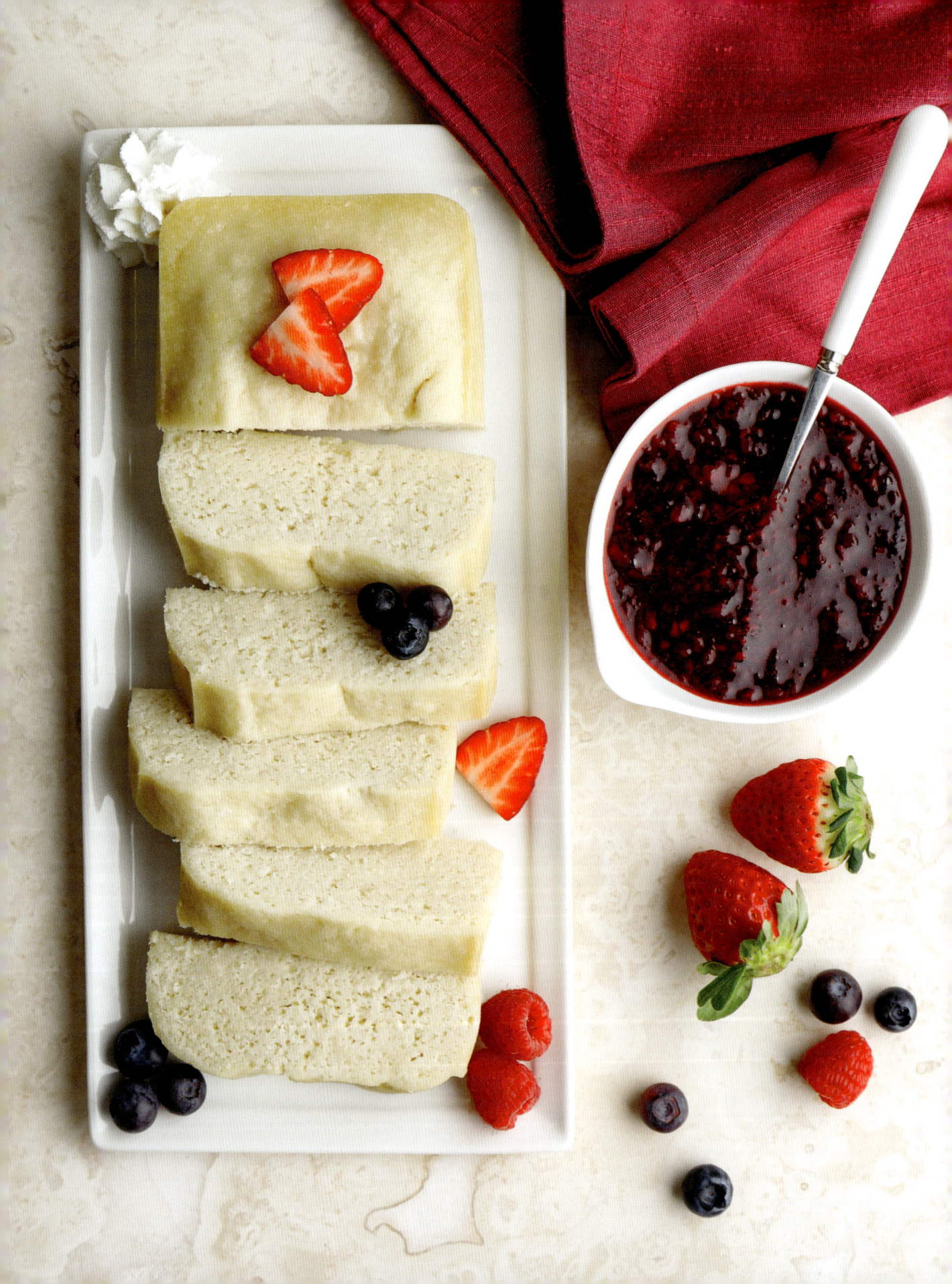

Prep Time: 10 min | High Pressure: 45 min | Natural Release: 10 min | Serves: 8

# Angel Bar Cake

We're not going to lie: when we first tried making this, we were really hoping it would rise higher, as our almond flour desserts typically do in the oven. When that didn't happen, we were ready to give up on making a low-carb cake—until we tasted it! The texture of this cake is so light and almost creamy; it's like a store-bought angel food or pound cake that melts in your mouth. It wasn't what we were intending to make but it may just be something better.

## Ingredients

Nonstick cooking spray
1 1/2 cups almond flour
2/3 cup sugar substitute
1 1/2 teaspoons baking powder
4 large egg whites
4 tablespoons butter, melted
1/4 cup heavy cream
1 1/2 teaspoons vanilla extract

## Special Equipment

6.5-inch loaf pan
Steam rack

1. Pour 1 cup of water into the Instant Pot. Spray a 6.5-inch loaf pan with nonstick cooking spray.

2. In a mixing bowl, combine almond flour, sugar substitute, and baking powder.

3. In a separate mixing bowl, whisk together egg whites, butter, heavy cream, and vanilla extract until egg whites are frothy.

4. Fold the wet ingredients into the dry ingredients to create a cake batter.

5. Spread the batter into the prepared loaf pan and tap against the counter to even out the top. Wrap bottom and all sides of the loaf pan in aluminum foil to prevent any water from seeping in. Place wrapped loaf pan on steam rack and carefully lower into the water bath in the Instant Pot.

6. Lock lid in place and seal pressure release vent. Set cooker to HIGH pressure for 45 minutes.

7. Let pressure release naturally for 10 minutes before opening the vent to let out any remaining pressure.

8. Let cool on counter for at least 30 minutes before refrigerating at least 2 hours. Slice and serve alongside fresh berries and sugar-free whipped cream, if desired.

### Instant Tips

This is also delicious when made with 1 teaspoon of coconut extract in place of 1 teaspoon of the vanilla extract. The texture of the cake is almost like the inside of an Almond Joy.

Calories: 220 | Fat: 19g | Protein: 6.5g | Total Carbs: 7g - Fiber: 2.5g = Net Carbs: 4.5g

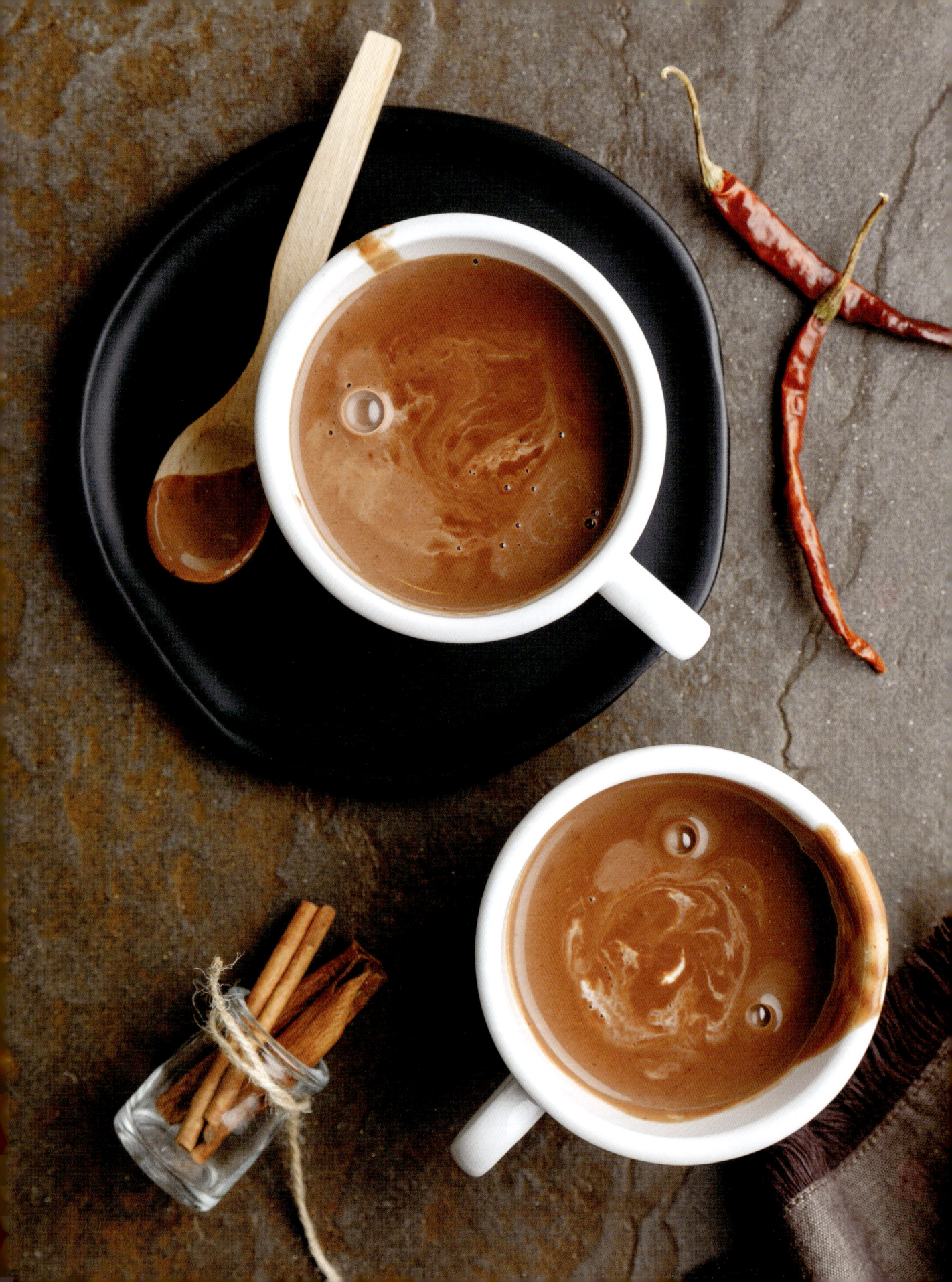

Prep Time: 5 min | High Pressure: 0 min | Natural Release: 15 min | Serves: 6

# Mexican Hot Chocolate

Cooking this hot chocolate in the Instant Pot allows you to infuse the flavor of cinnamon and heat of cayenne. For a party or gathering, you can even set the cooker to WARM to keep the cocoa ready all night long.

## Ingredients

2 cups unsweetened almond milk
1 cup water
1/2 cup sugar substitute
1/3 cup unsweetened cocoa powder
1/2 teaspoon vanilla extract
1/8 teaspoon cayenne pepper
1 cinnamon stick
1 cup heavy cream
Sugar-free whipped cream, to top

1. In the Instant Pot, whisk together almond milk, water, sugar substitute, cocoa powder, vanilla extract, and cayenne pepper.

2. Stir in cinnamon stick.

3. Lock lid in place and seal pressure release vent. Set cooker to HIGH pressure for 0 minutes.

4. Let pressure release naturally for 15 minutes before opening vent to let out remaining pressure.

5. Stir in heavy cream before serving topped with whipped cream.

### Instant Tips

The cayenne pepper adds a spicy kick to the hot chocolate but can be omitted if that isn't desired.

Calories: 170 | Fat: 16.5g | Protein: 2g | Total Carbs: 6g - Fiber: 2g = Net Carbs: 4g

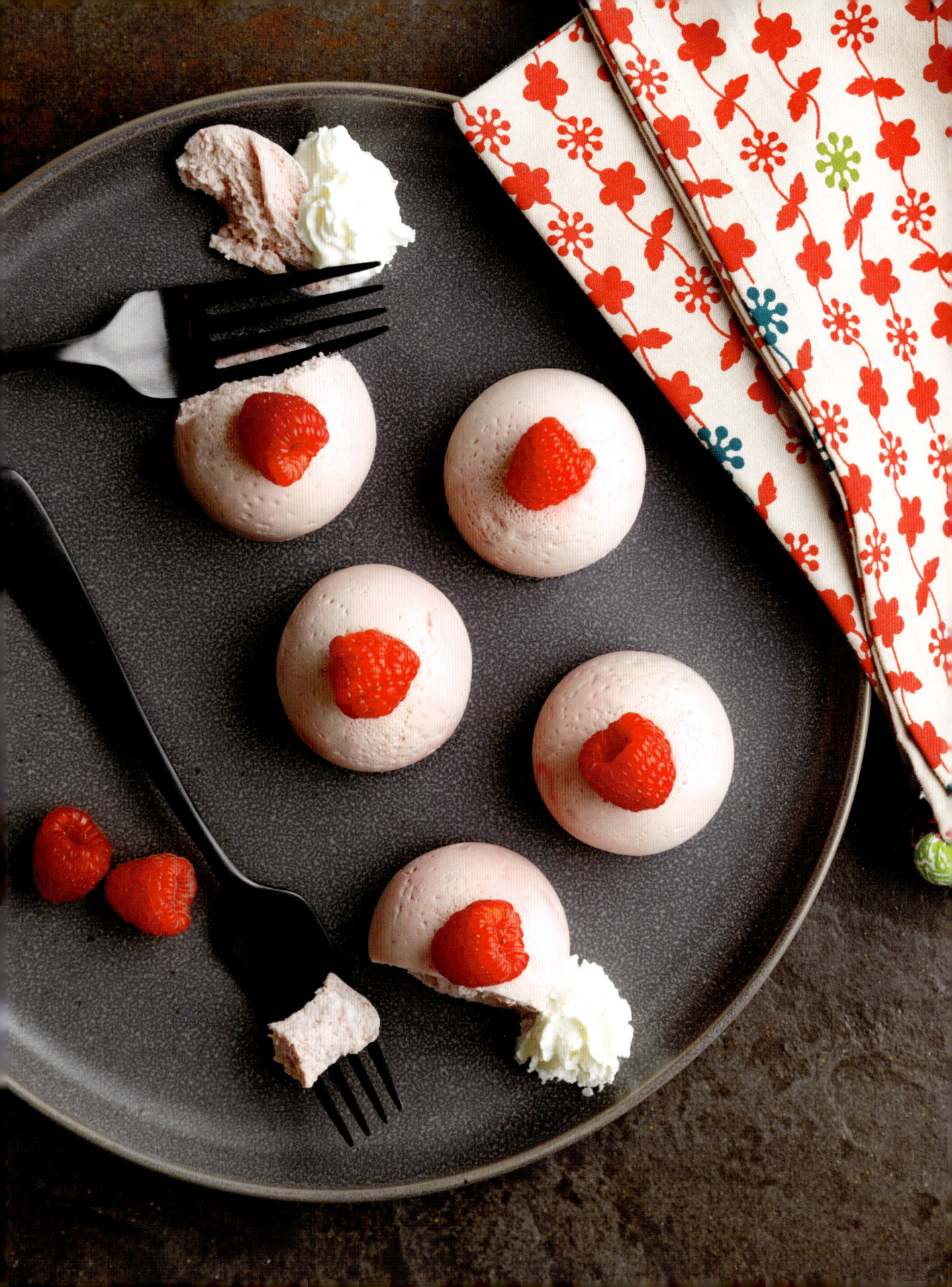

Prep Time: 10 min | High Pressure: 12 min | Natural Release: 15 min | Serves: 7

# Raspberry Cheesecake Bites

Just because it is an "egg bites mold" doesn't mean it is limited to only making egg bites! Here we've used the mold to make miniature cheesecakes with fresh raspberries puréed right into the batter.

## Ingredients

Nonstick cooking spray
¼ cup fresh raspberries
8 ounces cream cheese
1 large egg
1 large egg yolk
⅓ cup sugar substitute
3 tablespoons heavy cream
¼ teaspoon vanilla extract

## Special Equipment

Egg bites mold
Steam rack

1. For best results, start with raspberries, cream cheese, eggs, and heavy cream at room temperature.
2. Pour 1 cup of water into the Instant Pot. Spray egg bites mold with nonstick cooking spray.
3. Place raspberries in a food processor and top with all remaining ingredients. Process just until smooth, with raspberries almost entirely puréed.
4. Evenly pour the batter into each cup of the egg bites mold. Tap the mold against the counter to remove any air bubbles before wrapping with aluminum foil.
5. Place egg bites mold on steam rack and lower into the water bath in the cooker.
6. Lock lid in place and seal pressure release vent. Set cooker to HIGH pressure for 12 minutes.
7. Let pressure release naturally for 15 minutes before opening vent to release any remaining pressure.
8. Cool on counter for at least 30 minutes, then chill at least 2 hours before popping out of mold to serve.

### Instant Tips

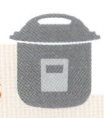

For a more vibrant pink color, we like to add 4 drops of red food coloring to the batter. It's purely a cosmetic choice with no impact on flavor.

Calories: 175 | Fat: 16.5g | Protein: 4g | Total Carbs: 3g - Fiber: 0.5g = Net Carbs: 2.5g

*Desserts*

Instant Low Carb • 217

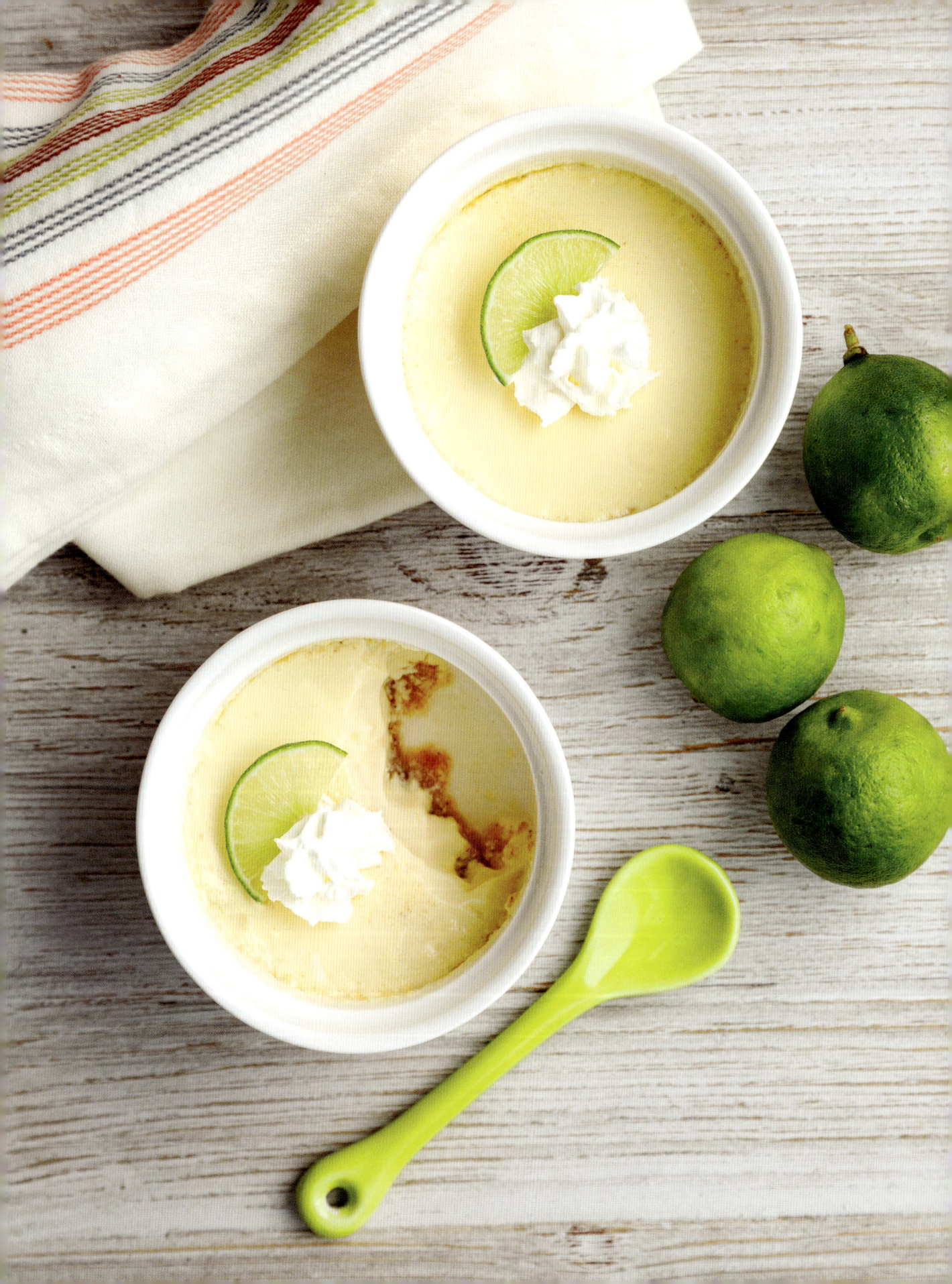

Prep Time: 15 min | High Pressure: 6 min | Natural Release: 5 min | Serves: 4

# Key Lime Custard Cups

These creamy Key Lime Custard Cups have a soft almond flour crust with just a hint of cinnamon to replicate the graham cracker crusts of traditional Key lime pie. As there are no high-carb starches or white sugar, the final consistency is closer to a pudding than firmer Key lime pie but is just as delicious.

## Ingredients

### Crust

¼ cup almond flour
1 tablespoon butter, melted
1 tablespoon sugar substitute
⅛ teaspoon ground cinnamon

### Filling

¾ cup heavy cream
¼ cup unsweetened almond milk
⅓ cup + 1 tablespoon sugar substitute
¼ teaspoon vanilla extract
3 large egg yolks
3 tablespoons Key lime juice
Sugar-free whipped cream

### Special Equipment

4 ramekins
Steam rack

### Instant Tips

Key lime juice is often sold in bottles near the fruit juice in the grocery store but also sometimes can be found in the produce section.

1. Pour 1 cup of water into the Instant Pot.

2. Use a fork to whisk together all Crust ingredients before pressing tightly into the bottom of 4 ramekins. You do not need to cover the entire bottom of the ramekin with the crust, only a large portion of the bottom.

3. In a saucepot on the stove set to medium heat, whisk together heavy cream, almond milk, sugar substitute, and vanilla extract. Whisking occasionally, bring up to a low simmer and immediately remove from heat.

4. Meanwhile, in a mixing bowl, whisk the egg yolks together. While whisking constantly, slowly pour the hot cream into the egg yolk mixture until combined.

5. Whisk the lime juice into the cream and egg mixture. For the best presentation, use a spoon to skim off any foam from the top of the mixture.

6. Pouring slowly as to not disturb the crust, divide the mixture evenly between the 4 ramekins and cover with aluminum foil. Place on steam rack and lower into the water bath in the cooker.

7. Lock lid in place and seal pressure release vent. Set cooker to HIGH pressure for 6 minutes.

8. Let pressure release naturally for 5 minutes before opening vent to let out remaining pressure.

9. Let cool on counter for at least 30 minutes before refrigerating at least 3 hours. Serve chilled, topped with whipped cream, if desired.

---

Calories: 280 | Fat: 26.5g | Protein: 4.5g | Total Carbs: 6.5g - Fiber: 1g = Net Carbs: 5.5g

# *Index*

**Artichokes**
Creamy Chicken with Artichokes, 107
Spinach with Artichokes, 150
Whole Artichokes, 49

**Asparagus**
Asparagus and Smoked Gouda Soup, 79
Lemon Pepper Asparagus, 185

**Avocado**
Shredded Chicken Burrito Bowls, 103
Southwestern Shirred Eggs, 31

**Bacon**
Beef Burgundy Soup, 83
Carbonara Brussels Sprouts, 197
Creamy Cauliflower and Ham Soup, 72
Maple Pecan Sprouts, 176
Quiche Lorraine, 33
Snap Peas with Crispy Pancetta, 158
Southern Collard Greens, 189
Tuscan Sausage Soup, 81

**Beef.** *See also* Ground Beef
Baby Back Ribs, 117
Balsamic Braised Short Ribs, 127
Barbacoa Beef, 119
Beef Burgundy Soup, 83
Beef Paprikash, 122
Beef Stroganoff, 129
Chuck Roast Chili, 69
Corned Beef and Cabbage, 139
Instant Pot Roast, 115
Italian Beef Stew, 78
Mongolian Beef, 135
Red Wine Braised Beef, 133
Steak and Eggplant Hash, 35
Sweet Onion Brisket, 126

**Berries**
Blueberry Muffin Cups, 41
Mixed Berry Sauce, 211
Raspberry Cheesecake Bites, 217
Really Good Iced Tea, 53

**Beverages**
Mexican Hot Chocolate, 215
Really Good Iced Tea, 53

**Breakfast.** *See also* Egg Dishes
Blueberry Muffin Cups, 41
Sausage and Sweet Potato Hash, 29
Steak and Eggplant Hash, 35

**Broccoli**
Broccoli Cheese Dip, 54
Broccoli Cheese Quiche, 39
Chicken Stir Fry, 99
Chicken with Broccoli Cheese Sauce, 109
Mongolian Beef, 135
Simply Steamed Broccoli, 195

**Brussels Sprouts**
Carbonara Brussels Sprouts, 197
Maple Pecan Sprouts, 176

**Cabbage**
Bratwurst with Honey Mustard Kraut, 121
Corned Beef and Cabbage, 139
Polish Sausage and Cabbage Soup, 77
Sweet-and-Sour Red Cabbage, 194

**Collard Greens**
Southern Collard Greens, 189

**Cauliflower, 17**
Butternut Squash Soup, 171
Cauliflower Fried Rice with Ham, 154
Cauliflower Risotto with Shrimp, 147
Chicken and Rice Soup, 82
Chicken and Shrimp Gumbo, 144
Creamy Cauliflower and Ham Soup, 72
Herb-Infused Mock Mashed Potatoes, 183
Instant Mock Mac and Cheese, 193
Shredded Chicken Burrito Bowls, 103
White "Bean" Dip with Pine Nuts, 59

## Chicken

Buffalo Wings, 47
Chicken and Rice Soup, 82
Chicken and Shrimp Gumbo, 144
Chicken Cacciatore, 111
Chicken Fajita Soup, 73
Chicken Marsala, 93
Chicken Noodle Soup, 67
Chicken Parmesan, 89
Chicken Sausage and Gouda Frittata, 28
Chicken Stir Fry, 99
Chicken Stock, 68
Chicken Verde, 96
Chicken with Broccoli Cheese Sauce, 109
Creamy Chicken with Artichokes, 107
Easier Cheesy Chili Chicken, 101
Family-Style Chicken Breasts, 104
Honey Mustard Chicken Drumsticks, 92
Indian Butter Chicken, 91
Margherita Chicken with Spaghetti Squash, 155
Orange Chicken, 108
Rotisserie-Style Chicken, 95
Shredded Chicken Burrito Bowls, 103
Sweet and Smoky Chicken Thighs, 100
Teriyaki Chicken Wings, 60

## Chocolate

Fudge Brownie Soufflé Cups, 209
Mexican Hot Chocolate, 215

## Cranberries

Cranberry Walnut Chutney, 167

## Desserts

Angel Bar Cake, 213
Cappuccino Flan, 207
Eggnog Cake with Bourbon Sauce, 177
Fudge Brownie Soufflé Cups, 209
Instant Cheesecake, 203
Key Lime Custard Cups, 219
Mexican Hot Chocolate, 215
Mixed Berry Sauce, 211
Orange and Cream Cheesecake Bites, 210
Peanut Pots de Crème, 205
Pumpkin Pie, 179
Raspberry Cheesecake Bites, 217

## Eggplant

Ratatouille, 199
Steak and Eggplant Hash, 35

## Eggs

Broccoli Cheese Quiche, 39
Chicken Sausage and Gouda Frittata, 28
Denver Egg Bites, 27
Instant Hard-Boiled Eggs, 61
Mushroom Swiss Coddled Eggs, 25
Pepperoni Pizza Egg Bites, 36
Perfect Poached Eggs, 37
Pimento-Cheese Deviled Eggs, 63
Quiche Lorraine, 33
Southwestern Shirred Eggs, 31
Spinach and Goat Cheese Egg Cups, 32

## Green Beans

Casserole-Style Green Beans, 175
Green Beans with Ham, 191
Marinated Green Bean Antipasto, 55

## Ground Beef

Cheesy Ground Beef Skillet, 159
Chipotle Chili, 75

## Ham

Cauliflower Fried Rice with Ham, 154
Creamy Cauliflower and Ham Soup, 72
Denver Egg Bites, 27
Green Beans with Ham, 191
Holiday Ham, 168
Marinated Green Bean Antipasto, 55
Swiss Chard with Prosciutto and Pine Nuts, 187

## Holiday Cooking

Butternut Squash Soup, 171
Casserole-Style Green Beans, 175
Cinnamon and Sage Pork Tenderloin, 172
Cranberry Walnut Chutney, 167
Eggnog Cake with Bourbon Sauce, 177
Holiday Ham, 168
Maple Pecan Sprouts, 176
Pumpkin Pie, 179
Sausage Stuffing, 169
Tender Turkey Breast, 165
Zesty Kale with Pistachios, 173

**Kale**
Creamed Kale, 190
Italian Sausage with Peppers and Kale, 132
Tuscan Sausage Soup, 81
Zesty Kale with Pistachios, 173

**Meats.** See also Beef; Pork
Greek Lamb Roast, 123

**Mushrooms**
Beef Burgundy Soup, 83
Beef Stroganoff, 129
Cheesy Ground Beef Skillet, 159
Chicken Cacciatore, 111
Chicken Marsala, 93
Chicken Stir Fry, 99
Cream of Mushroom Soup, 71
Greek Marinated Mushrooms, 51
Instant Pot Roast, 115
Mushroom Swiss Coddled Eggs, 25
Sausage Stuffing, 169

**Nuts**
Boiled Peanuts, 57
Cranberry Walnut Chutney, 167
Indian-Spiced Cashews, 157
Maple Pecan Sprouts, 176
Peanut Pots de Crème, 205
Pumpkin Pie, 179
Zesty Kale with Pistachios, 173

**Orange**
Orange and Cream Cheesecake Bites, 210
Orange Chicken, 108
Orange Ginger Edamame, 48

**Pine Nuts**
Swiss Chard with Prosciutto and Pine Nuts, 187
White "Bean" Dip with Pine Nuts, 59

**Pork.** See also Bacon; Ham; Sausage
Barbecue Pulled Pork, 125
Boneless Ribs with Sweet Chili Sauce, 136
Cinnamon and Sage Pork Tenderloin, 172
Jamaican Jerk Pork Shoulder, 118
Pork Carnitas, 137
Tequila Pork Tenderloin, 131

**Poultry.** See Chicken; Turkey

**Radishes**
Chicken Noodle Soup, 67
Instant Pot Roast, 115
Pickled Radishes, 45
Red Bliss Radishes, 161

**Sausage**
Bratwurst with Honey Mustard Kraut, 121
Chicken and Shrimp Gumbo, 144
Chicken Sausage and Gouda Frittata, 28
Italian Sausage with Peppers and Kale, 132
Marinated Green Bean Antipasto, 55
Polish Sausage and Cabbage Soup, 77
Sausage and Sweet Potato Hash, 29
Sausage Stuffing, 169
Tuscan Sausage Soup, 81

**Sauté**
Cauliflower Fried Rice with Ham, 154
Cauliflower Risotto with Shrimp, 147
Cheesy Ground Beef Skillet, 159
Chicken and Shrimp Gumbo, 144
Ground Turkey Bolognese, 151
Indian-Spiced Cashews, 157
Instant Popcorn, 153
Margherita Chicken with Spaghetti Squash, 155
Red Bliss Radishes, 161
Scallops with Capers and Dill, 149
Snap Peas with Crispy Pancetta, 158
Spinach with Artichokes, 150
Zucchini in Clam Sauce, 145

**Seafood**
Cauliflower Risotto with Shrimp, 147
Chicken and Shrimp Gumbo, 144
Scallops with Capers and Dill, 149
Simple Salmon Fillets with Dill, 143
Zucchini in Clam Sauce, 145

**Sides**
Carbonara Brussels Sprouts, 197
Casserole-Style Green Beans, 175
Cranberry Walnut Chutney, 167
Creamed Kale, 190
Green Beans with Ham, 191

**Sides,** *continued*
Herb-Infused Mock Mashed Potatoes, 183
Instant Mock Mac and Cheese, 193
Lemon Pepper Asparagus, 185
Maple Pecan Sprouts, 176
Ratatouille, 199
Sausage Stuffing, 169
Simply Steamed Broccoli, 195
Southern Collard Greens, 189
Spaghetti Squash, 186
Sweet-and-Sour Red Cabbage, 194
Swiss Chard with Prosciutto and Pine Nuts, 187
Zesty Kale with Pistachios, 173

**Soups**
Asparagus and Smoked Gouda Soup, 79
Beef Burgundy Soup, 83
Butternut Squash Soup, 171
Chicken and Rice Soup, 82
Chicken and Shrimp Gumbo, 144
Chicken Fajita Soup, 73
Chicken Noodle Soup, 67
Chicken Stock, 68
Chipotle Chili, 75
Chuck Roast Chili, 69
Cream of Mushroom Soup, 71
Creamy Cauliflower and Ham Soup, 72
Creamy Tomato Soup, 85
Italian Beef Stew, 78
Polish Sausage and Cabbage Soup, 77
Tuscan Sausage Soup, 81

**Spinach**
Spinach and Goat Cheese Egg Cups, 32
Spinach with Artichokes, 150

**Squash**
Beef Burgundy Soup, 83
Beef Stroganoff, 129
Butternut Squash Soup, 171
Cheesy Ground Beef Skillet, 159
Chicken Noodle Soup, 67
Ground Turkey Bolognese, 151
Italian Beef Stew, 78
Margherita Chicken with Spaghetti Squash, 155
Orange Chicken, 108
Ratatouille, 199
Spaghetti Squash, 186
Tuscan Sausage Soup, 81
Zucchini in Clam Sauce, 145

**Starters**
Boiled Peanuts, 57
Broccoli Cheese Dip, 54
Buffalo Wings, 47
Greek Marinated Mushrooms, 51
Indian-Spiced Cashews, 157
Instant Hard-Boiled Eggs, 61
Instant Popcorn, 153
Marinated Green Bean Antipasto, 55
Orange Ginger Edamame, 48
Pickled Radishes, 45
Pimento-Cheese Deviled Eggs, 63
Really Good Iced Tea, 53
Teriyaki Chicken Wings, 60
White "Bean" Dip with Pine Nuts, 59
Whole Artichokes, 49

**Sweet Potatoes**
Sausage and Sweet Potato Hash, 29

**Tomatoes**
Chicken and Shrimp Gumbo, 144
Chicken Cacciatore, 111
Chipotle Chili, 75
Chuck Roast Chili, 69
Creamy Chicken with Artichokes, 107
Creamy Tomato Soup, 85
Indian Butter Chicken, 91
Italian Beef Stew, 78
Ratatouille, 199

**Turkey**
Cajun Turkey Tenderloin, 105
Ground Turkey Bolognese, 151
Pepperoni Pizza Egg Bites, 36
"Roasted" Turkey Legs, 97
Tender Turkey Breast, 165

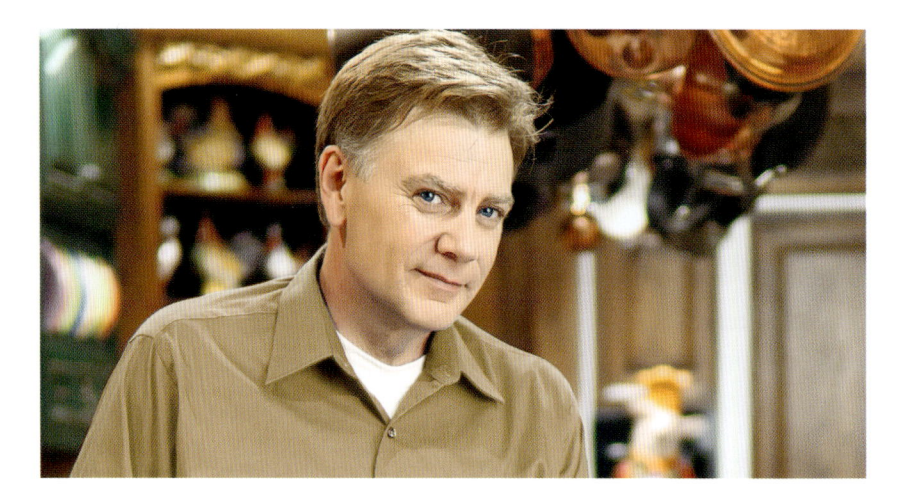

**George Stella** has been a professional chef for over 30 years. He has appeared on numerous television and news shows, including two seasons of his own show, ***Low Carb and Lovin' It***, on the Food Network. Most recently he appeared on *The Dr. Oz Show*.

Connecticut born, George has spent more than half of his life in Florida, where he lives today, with his wife, Rachel. This is his tenth cookbook.

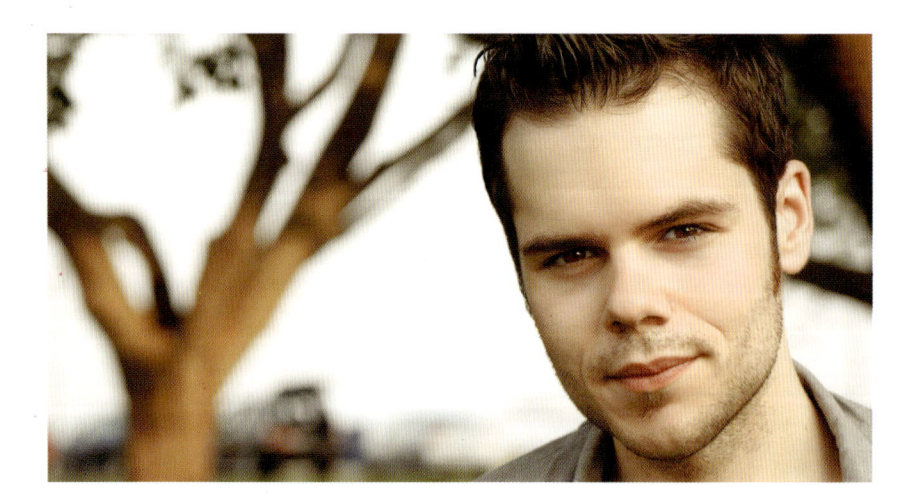

**Christian Stella** is a recipe developer and food photographer for product and food manufacturers. Along with his wife, Elise, he has worked on over forty food-related projects in the last decade. He is also an indie film director with his first major movie debuting later this year.